HONEST BEAUTY TALKS

Crystal Gua Sha Facials & other Holistic Beauty Rituals.

Written by Maja Lemmeke Hansen & Tanja Eskildsen
Graphic design: Laila Bunk
Translation: Sharon Bjørling

The conversation that started it all

Honest Beauty Talks originated from a conversation between Maja and Tanja. A conversation and an aspiration for a more honest and loving beauty industry. A wish that we, as women, learn to fill ourselves with self-loving rituals that give us an effect on both skin, body and mind.

We named it "Honest Beauty Talks".

We would like to invite you into our conversation through this book you now hold in your hands.

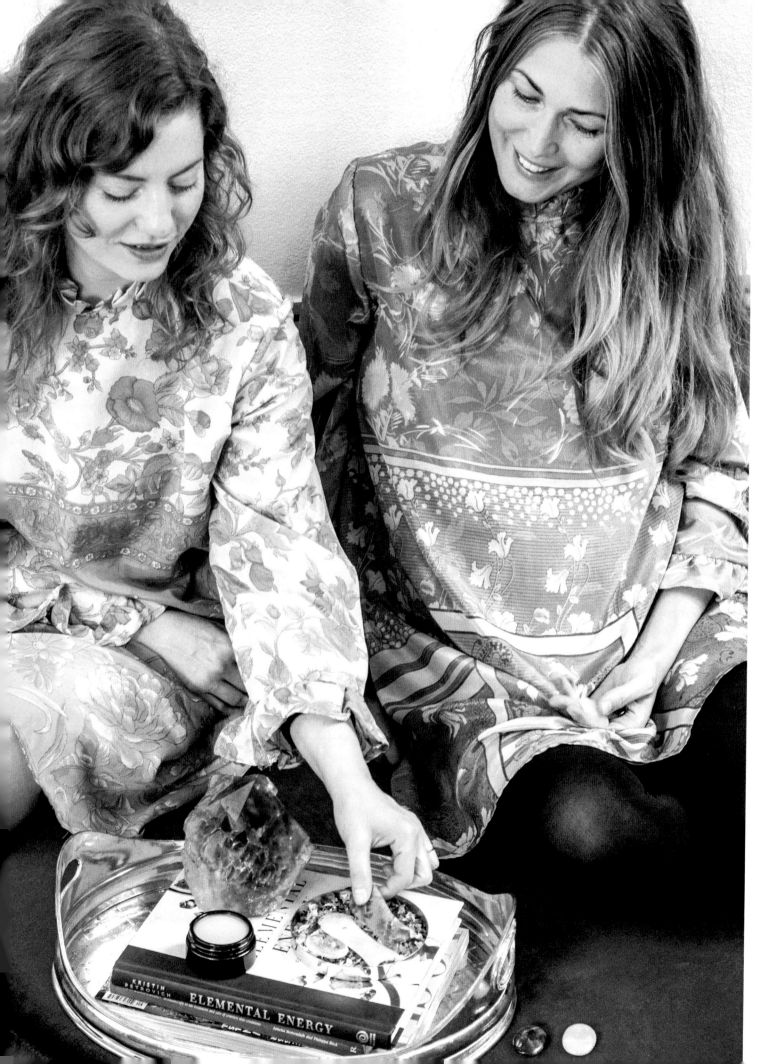

Content

1

06   HONEST BEAUTY TALKS
10   Holistic Beauty
12   How to use this book

2

14   COLLABORATE WITH YOUR SKIN
20   Skin Cycle
22   Hormonal Cycle of the Skin
24   Hormonal Breakouts

3

28   CRYSTAL ENERGY
32   Amethyst
34   Clear Quartz
36   Aventurine
38   Sodalite
40   Rose Quartz
42   Cleanse your Crystals

4

44   WHY IS GUA SHA A HIT?

5

52   DIY SKINCARE
54   Creating Beauty through the Science of Scent
58   Bestseller Facebalms
58   How to make the perfect facebalm
60   Calmness recipe
62   Self-Love recipe
64   Trust recipe
66   Clarity recipe
68   Freedom recipe
70   Multi-purpose Facebalm
71   How to use the Facebalm

Content

6

72 BODY GUA SHA
74 Scrape away your Cellulite
77 What you need to get started
78 How fit is your fascia?
79 Cellulite scheme
80 The 4 types of Cellulite
81 Draw your cellulite types
82 Body Gua Sha Massage
82 Body Gua Sha Techniques
83 Body Gua Sha - Time overview
85 Gua Sha FAQ
86 Body Detoxbalm

7

88 GUA SHA FACIALS
90 A Good Start
92 Puffy Face
94 Sensitive Skin
96 Pimples
98 Eye Lift
100 Worry Lines
102 Jaw Tension
104 Mouth & Lips
106 Neck & Jawline
108 Scar Tissue & Wrinkles
110 Cheek Lift

8

112 STAY IN TOUCH
114 Disclaimer

Honest Beauty Talks

We dream of a world where beauty emerges from pleasure and well-being. A world where beauty is defined by self-worth and love for oneself.

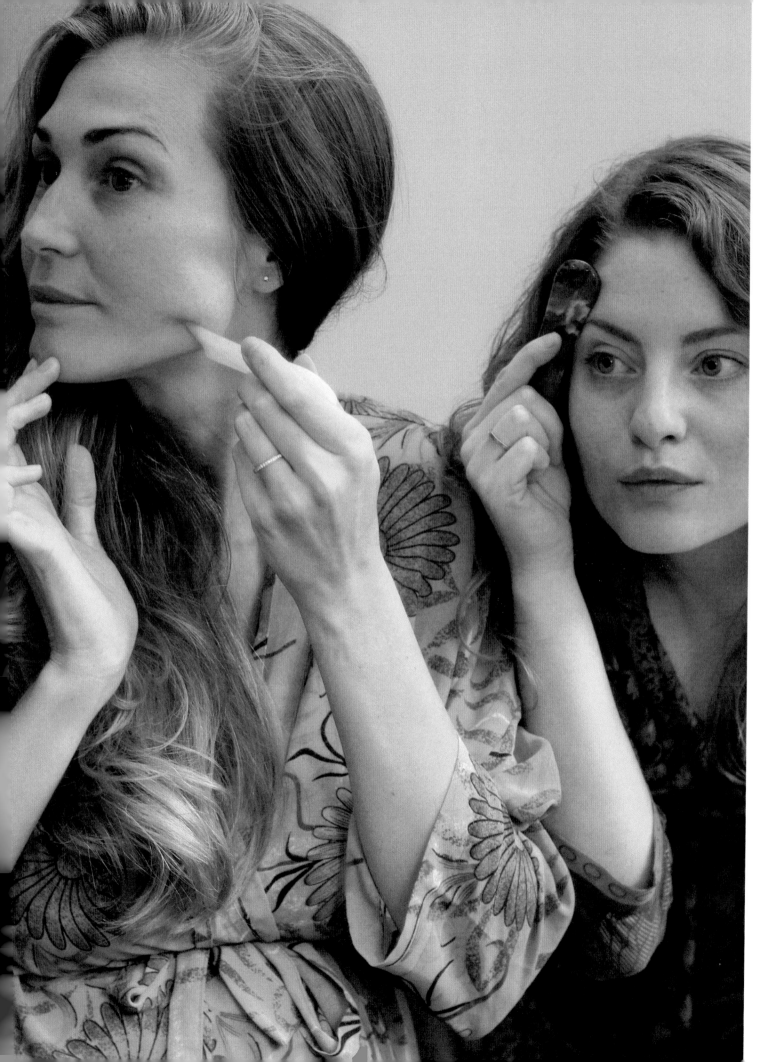

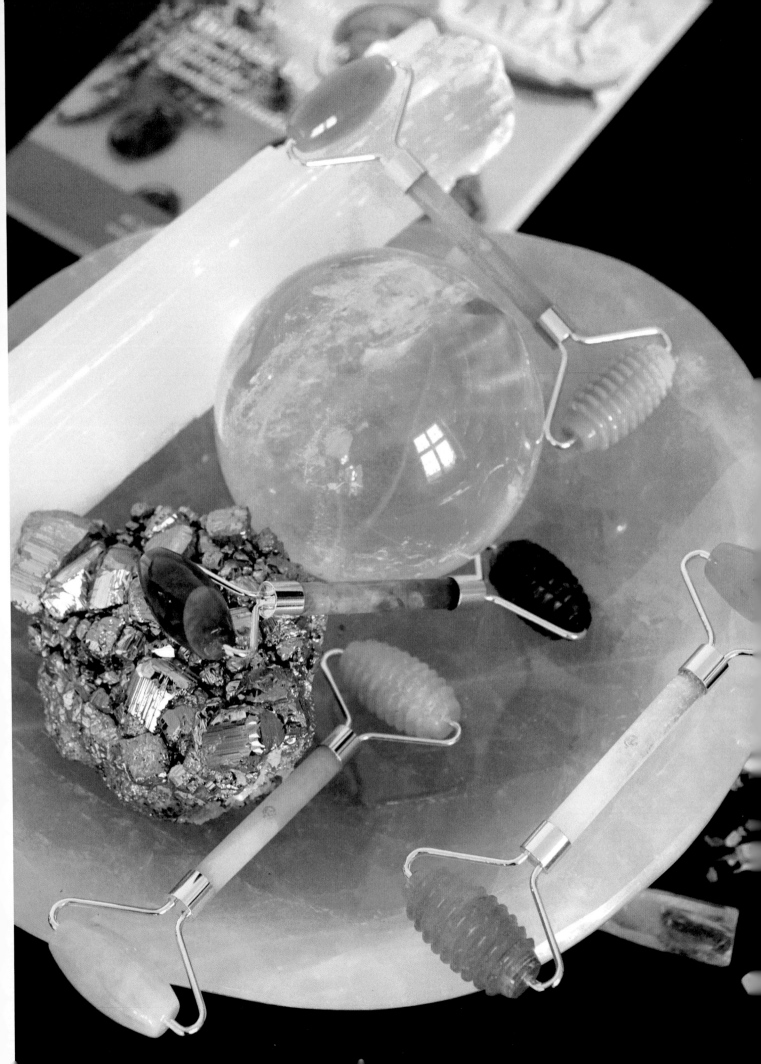

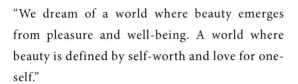

"We dream of a world where beauty emerges from pleasure and well-being. A world where beauty is defined by self-worth and love for oneself."

Currently, we feel that we live in a world where beauty has lost its authenticity and integrity is something we really yearn for. We live in a world of manipulated models and with filters on our everyday lives. This leads to a distorted view of beauty and we lose ourselves in the struggle to strive to look like something that isn't real. And that is a stressful beauty paradigm to live in!

True beauty is defined by self awareness, self worth & self love

It was the conversation about the connection between skin problems and chronic stress that lead us to create Honest Beauty Talks in the first place.

In 2015 we set out with a dream of creating a beauty product that could stimulate the relaxation response through the senses of touch and smell.

We combined our love for crystals and healing aromatherapy with our favorite massage techniques to give you a modern, luxurious yet simple version of gua sha facials.

Our DIY facials gives you a well-deserved break in your everyday life whilst caring for your skin and mind.

We believe in beauty rituals that create harmony through balancing the body's energy system, lymphatic system, nervous system and hormone system. Thus, creating a healthy foundation where beauty can manifest itself.

Our DIY Crystal Gua Sha Facials are designed to work on your exterior beauty and inner health while giving you a "break" in your everyday life. Gua Sha massage gives a sense of presence and tranquility, so you are more capable of feeling and listening to your body. We believe this leads to a greater satisfaction and well-being in your life.

We have designed several different Gua Sha beauty tools and accompanying DIY face balm kits, so you can create the one ritual that fits your "personality" and skin type the best.

If you need any guidance we are always here to help. Reach out to care@honestbeautytalks.org

Holistic Beauty

Why we work with holistic beauty.

In today's society where stress has become a major part of our everyday lives, we see a great need to create rituals that help the body back into balance.

WHAT IS STRESS?

The experience of stress occurs when the demands made to us, exceed our (perceived) ability to manage them. Stress can be defined as changes in our mental, emotional and physical state, due to demands outside and inside ourselves. It is of course important to mention that stress itself is not a bad thing. It is a necessity for survival and helps us to find the balance between action and being. The problem arises when stress becomes chronic and we either end up in a state of sympathetic dominance, or even worse parasympathetic dominance.

How does stress affect your skin, body and cells?

1 When you are in a state of stress, all your energy is used to protect your vital organs.

2 Contraction of the blood vessels.

3 Restriction in blood flow in the skin´s small capillaries.

4 The skin is starved of nourishment and cannot eliminate waste.

5 Inflammation occurs which breaks down collagen and connective tissue, causing the cells to "caramelize".

6 This results in sagging and rigid skin tissue that cannot retain moisture.

You may have experienced this; your skin goes berserk in periods when you are too busy or have too much on your mind. It may appear on the skin as inflammation, dryness, impurities, redness, etc.

When the sympathetic nervous system is triggered, the body is placed in a state of increased alertness, setting off a cascade of physiological changes that influence muscle strength, the immune system and the circulation. The parasympathetic nervous system, on the other hand, combats the "fight or flight" mechanism and initiates digestion; thereby, maintaining and building the body.

When the skin reacts, it is not because there is something wrong with your skin. The skin responds, as it is biologically programmed to do, when something is off. Your skin tries to connect with you, through symptoms, by showing you a reflection of something being off balance.

BEAUTY IS IN YOUR HANDS.

Your task is now to take responsibility for your skin and listen to what your body is trying to tell you. We promise you, that if you really start listening to your body, you can create nothing less than miracles.

Your body has self-healing powers. There is more and more scientific evidence that proves how external lifestyle factors such as nutrition, environment, exercise, positive or negative thinking patterns and emotions literally affect our DNA.

So, what has this got to do about stress? Your body produces many different hormones which are essential for the human body. The problem, however, arises when there is an imbalance in hormones. For example, if you get too many stress hormones in the body.

When the body is exposed to a potential threat, it activates the sympathetic nervous system. Which is not a bad thing, it just means that your body is preparing for battle. Unfortunately, the reptilian brain does not distinguish between a threat that is life-threatening or just a thought that triggers the stress response because of negative thoughts, stress at work or family problems, etc. The problem occurs if you constantly activate your stress response throughout the day.

So, as long as your stress response is activated, the body does not deal with long-term problems like cell renewal, self- reparation and skin aging. Instead, it´s in full swing, fighting for survival and extinguishing acute fires in the body. When the inflammation becomes chronic, it may so-metimes appear in a variety of skin problems, and eventually result in disease. If you experience a skin problem for the first time, do not ignore it and listen to what your body is trying to tell you.

We are not saying that this applies to all skin problems. But many are stress related and a calm, well-balanced body is more equipped to fight bacteria and virus than a stressed out one. The recipe is simple. You need to activate the relaxation response through the parasympathetic nervous system. And it responds to CARING TOUCH. Not just from others but from your own loving hands.

What we've learned, in our work, as a cosmetologist and holistic skin therapist, over the past 10 years, is that it takes hard work to treat the symptoms and it never gives a complete satisfactory result. Instead, the solution is to put more energy into what we do to explore and identify the underlying cause of the ”problem” so we can prevent it from happening again. Unfortunately, we are very sorry to reveal that we do not find the solution is in a cream or quick fix.

"We achieve the best results by having a balanced energy system. a strong nervous system. happy hormones. a healthy diet. a positive mind and a lot of nurturing self-love"

How to use this book

- This book is for you who believe in natural non-invasive alternative to effective skin care

- This book is for you who longs to treat the cause, not the symptom

- This book is for you with a skin condition you wish to solve

- This book is for you who wants to add radiance to your skin

- This book is for you who wants to keep wrinkles at bay without any side effects

- This book is for you who wants to reduce your stress level

- This book is for you who yearns for more inner wellbeing

P.S It is important that you are aware and well informed about the contra-indications of a Gua Sha massage. Always seek the advice of your physician if you are in doubt.

THE BOOK IS DIVIDED INTO TWO PARTS
The theoretical section will give you an understanding of your skin, how it is submissive to a natural cycle and the self-healing properties it possesses. This section also gives you knowledge about the origins of Gua Sha massage and how it works.

The practical part teaches you how to prepare for the Gua Sha massage. We will teach you how to make your own natural skin care products and facebalms, customized to your skin type and designed for the perfect gua sha facial treatment. You will learn to perform 10 DIY crystal Gua Sha Facials and 1 for the body. We have included several holistic skin tips for different skin problems, that will help you reach your goals faster.

Although it is tempting to go straight to the practical part, we recommend that you embark on your Gua Sha journey in a slow and deliberate manner by introducing the theoretical part first. That way, we are confident that you are" well equipped "and motivated before you begin the practical part. The practical part is designed to help you with certain skin problems that might pertain to you.

If you have questions concerning the book and our crystal Gua Sha massage, please feel free to write to us at our mail: care@honestbeautytalks.org or join our Facebook group: Honest Beauty Talks. You can also find our video for the DIY facials on our website www.honestbeautytalks.com.

We wish you all the best with your new beauty ritual!

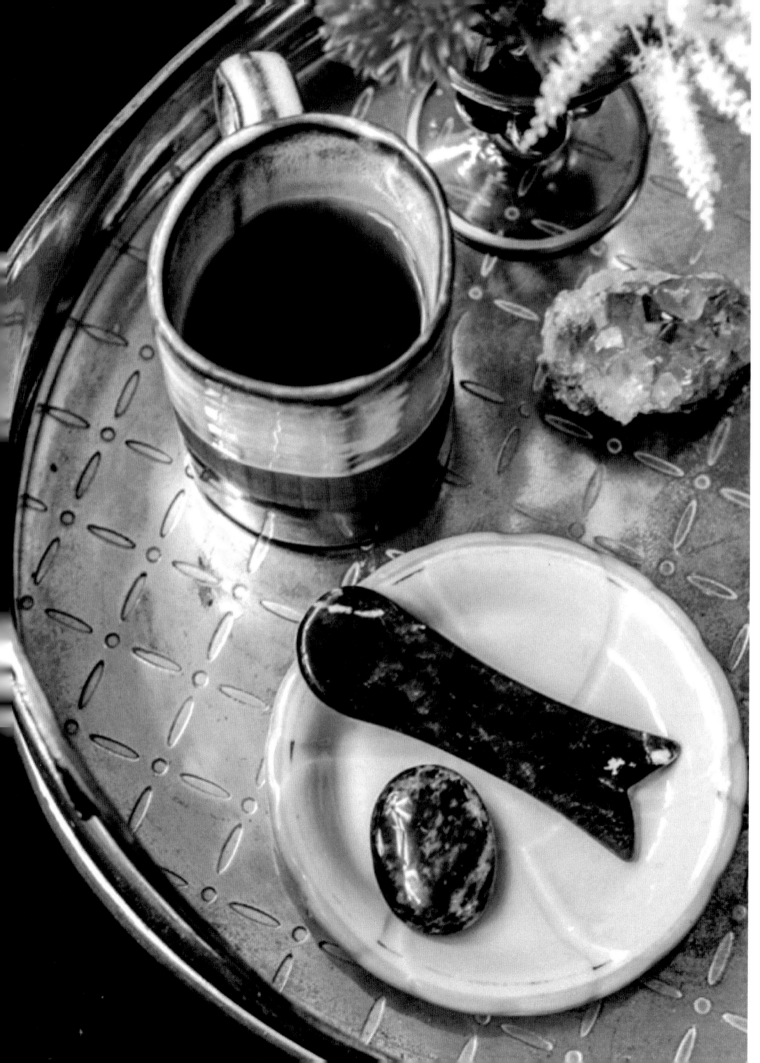

Collaborate with your SKIN

Do you work with or against your skin? Knowing the natural cycle of your skin with its biological rhythm and self-healing properties, will give you faster results.

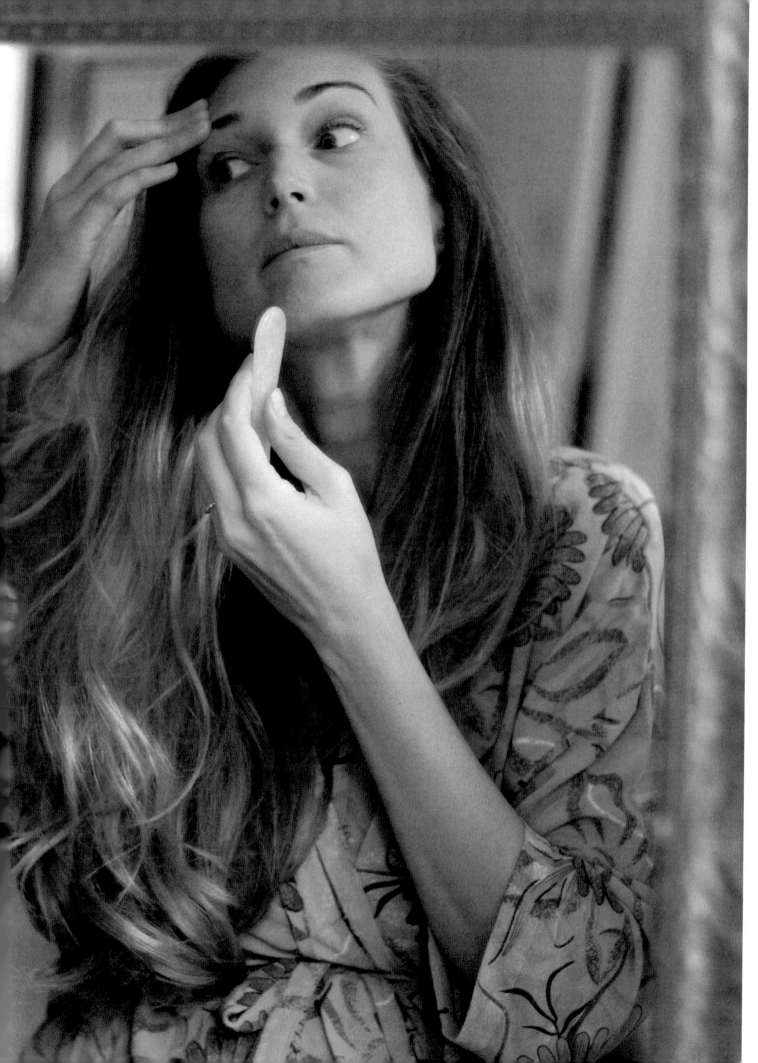

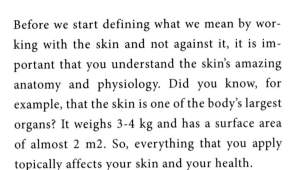

Before we start defining what we mean by working with the skin and not against it, it is important that you understand the skin's amazing anatomy and physiology. Did you know, for example, that the skin is one of the body's largest organs? It weighs 3-4 kg and has a surface area of almost 2 m2. So, everything that you apply topically affects your skin and your health.

The thickness of the skin varies from 0.05 mm, on thinnest skin like the eyelids, up to 5 mm or more in places where it is particularly exposed to severe pressure, such as the soles of the feet. The skin is the fastest tissue to regenerate in the body, but it is also the last to receive nutrition.

Every month, the outermost layer, called the epidermis, is replaced completely. This occurs at a rapid rate of about 30,000 cell divisions per minute. Therefore, you won´t typically know if a new skin care regimen is working for you until at least a month. This is all good advice, but the reality is, unfortunately, a bit more complex. You see, the skin reflects our whole body, not just dietary habits, skin care routines and lifestyle, but also our emotional and hormonal (in) balance.

The skin's vulnerable and exposed position, plus dynamic and responsive nature makes the skin change appearance frequently over a lifetime. indeed, the skin may change appearance several times in just one day! Changes in the skin, may be due to exposure to harmful chemical substances (eg in skin care), radiation damage from UV light, radioactivity and internal stress (eg emotional stress or poor diet).

Our skin is more than just a passive waterproof protective layer covering our body. It is an extremely complex, interactive and impressive body, built by many specialized cells.

The epidermis, the outermost layer of skin, provides a protective waterproof barrier. It is this layer we primarily treat with skin care.

The dermis, beneath the epidermis, contains connective tissue, sebaceous glands, sweat glands and blood vessels that affect not only the appearance of the skin, but also the skin's nutrient absorption and excretion.

Under dermis, lies the deeper subcutaneous tissue, hypodermis, made of fat and connective tissue. This can either give skin a full look or a slim look, depending on the condition of the subcutaneous insulating lipid layer and collagen structure. Dermis is the primary skin layer we want to influence with the Gua Sha massage.

Dermis consists mainly of connective tissue and primarily gives the skin firmness and elasticity. Dermis varies in thickness from 0.3 mm on the eyelid to 3.0 mm on the back. Dermis has two layers:
1) The top papillary layer that contains a thin structure of collagen fibers.
2) The lower reticular layer, which is thicker and made of densely packed collagen fibers.

Dermis contains a rich network of blood vessels which partly provide dermis and epidermis with oxygen and nutrition, and partly provide important functions in connection with temperature regulation, sensory function and the skin immune system.

Dermis's structure consists of:

- connective tissue
- elastin fibers
- fibroblasts
- sebaceous glands
- sweat glands
- lymphatic capillaries
- blood vessels/capillaries
- hair follicles
- sensory nerve endings

Connective tissue

Connective tissue contains fibroblasts which produce an extracellular matrix; a structural framework outside the cells. This is composed of water-binding substances such as hyaluronic acid and chondroitin sulfates (GAGS). These produce a gel, in which the fibers in the connective tissue are embedded. The tissue fibers, which are constructed of collagen and elastin, give the connective tissues mechanical durability. Connective tissue consists of elastin and collagen, which help to give skin its strength, elasticity and flexibility.

Skin nutrition for connective tissue

Protein and vitamin C are the building blocks for healthy collagen. GAGS supplementation and sufficient fluid provide a healthy and moisturized connective tissue. In addition, you can eat Bone Broth or collagen powder along with flavonoids from e.g. rosehip powder to give the connective tissue an extra boost. Abstain from sugar and starches as they contribute to glucosylation of the connective tissue which makes it rigid and inflexible.

Elastin fibers

As the name suggests, the elastin fibers give the skin elasticity and flexibility.

Skin nutrition for elastin fibers

Protein, liquid, Vitamin C, GAGS.

Fibroblasts

Fibroblasts produce collagen, which is important for wound healing and skin firmness. Collagen strengthens and support the skin's structure. Collagen also provides wound and scar healing properties.

Skin nutrition for fibroblasts

Protein, Liquid, Vitamin C, GAGS.

Sebaceous glands

Sebaceous glands secrete sebum, which consists of triglycerides, wax esters, squalene, free fatty acids, salts and lactic acid. Sebum maintains the skin's pH between 4.5 and 6, keeping skin and hair healthy, thus protecting against bacteria and dehydration. Sebum ensures that the skin's barrier is waterproof.

Skin nutrition for the sebaceous glands

The production of sebum is influenced by insulin, cortisol and testosterone. Relaxation, as well as a blood sugar stabilizing diet, help regulate sebum production.

Sweat glands

The sweat glands produce sweat to regulate body temperature. Apocrine glands are found almost exclusively in the armpit and secrete a thicker sweat, especially when nervous or stressed. The sweat glands help regulate the body temperature and the excretion of minerals and waste products.

Skin nutrition for the sweat glands
Hot spices such as ginger, elderflower and chili exacerbate sweat production. Sage tea reduces perspiration.

Lymphatic capillaries
The lymphatic capillaries remove excess fluid, that leaks into the tissue, and brings it back to the bloodstream. Lymphatic fluid contains white blood cells which play a role in the immune system. The lymph makes sure that bacteria, toxins and other foreign bodies are destroyed and excreted so that they don´t accumulate in the body.

Skin nutrition for the lymph
The lymphatic system is compromised by poor circulation and lack of oxygen (insufficient breathing and lack of exercise). Tea and extract from echinacea, marigold and linden flower stimulate the lymphatic circulation, and so do exercise, massage, cold baths, sauna, deep breathing, Gua Sha and dry brushing.

Blood vessels
Blood vessels in the dermis deliver nourishment to, and remove waste products from, the cells in the epidermis. The epidermis does not have blood vessels and therefore no direct blood flow. The blood vessels can expand or constrict to regulate body temperature. The blood vessels provide nutritional support for the regeneration of cells in the basal (deepest) layer and provide temperature regulation.

Skin nutrition for blood vessels
The blood vessels are compromised by weak blood circulation, lack of oxygen (insufficient breathing and exercise). Exercise, massage, cold baths, sauna, deep breathing, Gua Sha and dry brushing strengthen the circulation and the blood vessels. Ginger, turmeric, astaxanthin, ginkgo biloba, white tuna and omega 3 from fish oil also strengthen blood vessels and circulation.

Hair follicles
Hair follicles have a preprogrammed growth cycle, where hair growth is rested and renewed over a two-year period. Hair has a protective function against heat loss, dust particles and UV rays.

Skin nourishment for hair follicles
The hair is strengthened by B vitamins, nettle tea, tea and sprouts of fenugreek seeds, selenium, zinc and silicon and compromised by stress and poor nutrient absorption.

Sensory nerve endings
The sensory nerve endings detect pressure, pain and touch. They send a message to the brain telling whether something is pleasurable or dangerous, and whether the brain should produce "happiness hormones" or stress hormones. The sensory nervous system tells us if the outside world is safe or dangerous.

Skin´s Self-Renewal Process
The deepest layer of the epidermis is constantly renewed by a process of cell division, called desquamation, which is responsible for the generation of new epidermal skin cells. The deep basal layer consists of cells that constantly divide as they progressively move towards the surface, pushed upwards, by newly formed cells beneath them. As the cells ascend, they develop small tips that hold them close together. At the same time, they become flatter and fill up with a waterproof protein called keratin.

The Keratinization Process
Eventually, the skin cells die and are reduced to flattened scales, filled with densely packed keratin. Once the cells are keratinized on the surface, they form a durable layer resembling a solid brick wall. This hardened layer is shed during daily wear on the skin and is constantly replaced by cells from below. The journey, from the basal layer to the surface, takes about 4 weeks, and typically we shed about 0.5 kg of skin cells per year.

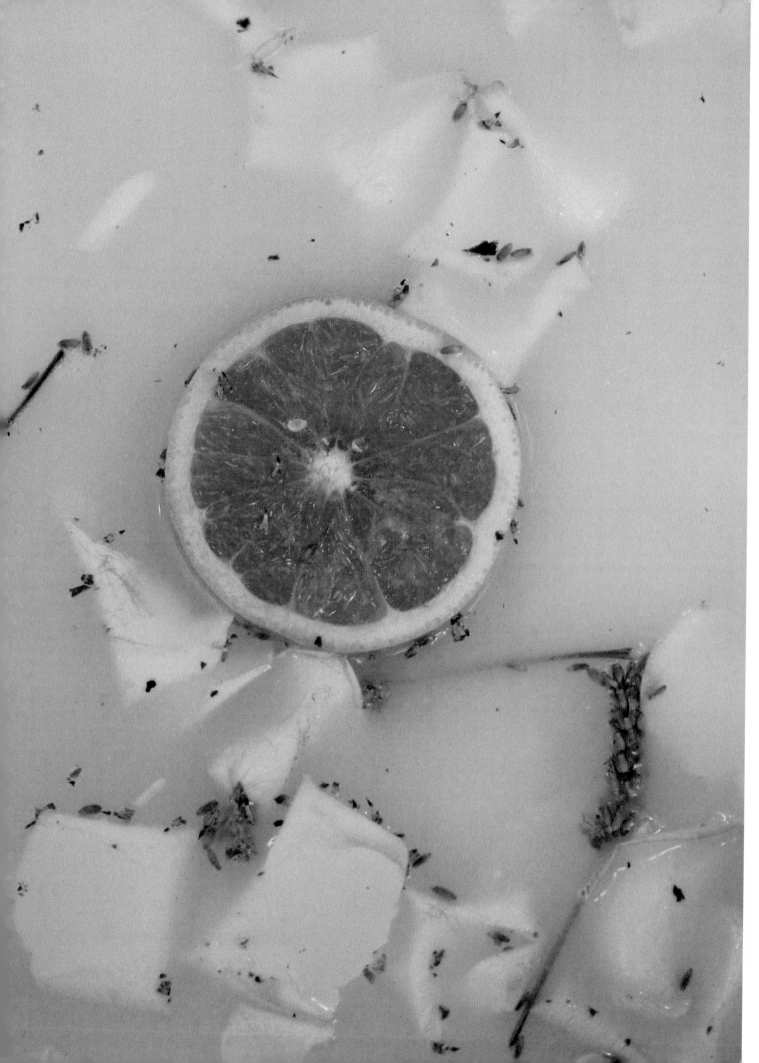

Skin Cycle

Do you work with or against your skin?

We can have the tendency to see normal skin changes as problems that need to be solved. But, if this were the case, it would be a full-time job because the skin follows a natural cycle that results in constant change in appearance.

We can do a lot to keep our skin healthy, but some things are beyond our control. The skin follows a daily rhythm and a monthly cycle, where it passes through different phases, that changes its appearance.

When you know the phases, you can plan your skin care routines, so that they work in harmony with the skin's natural cycle and thereby achieve better results.

THE DAILY RHYTHM OF THE SKIN

A normal healthy skin can change, almost instantly, from one hour to the next. On the following chart, you can follow the skin's natural daily cycle. This will give you a better idea of which products you should add to your skin, and at what times.

"We can have the tendency to see normal skin changes as problems that need to be solved. But, if this were the case, it would be a full-time job because the skin follows a natural cycle that results in constant change in appearance."

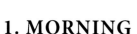

1. MORNING

You have a higher risk of getting an allergic reaction in the morning than in the afternoon.

8:00 A.M.

The skin is not nearly as receptive in the morning as it is in the afternoon, so it´s not a good idea to use nourishing masks and heavy creams / sera around this time.

Instead, support the skin by drinking a large glass of water with apple cider vinegar and possibly a cup of nettle tea.
Consume a blood sugar stabilizing breakfast with enough fats and fiber, as this has a calming effect on the nervo

2. AFTERNOON

The production of new skin cells is at its lowest around lunch, so here you can experience that skin problems like psoriasis are worse. Oil production is at its highest, so the skin may feel more greasy and appear shiny in the T-zone.

The most sustainable way to treat an overactive sebum production is to control stress levels and blood sugar. Be sure to eat blood sugar-friendly and get enough "calming" fats for breakfast and lunch.

4:00 P.M.

The skin is extra receptive to active ingredients around 4:00 p.m., so this is a good time for nourishing masks, sera and facial treatments.

3. EVENING

The skin is most balanced in the afternoon and evening. There is a greater risk of losing moisture at night, so use nourishing creams and sera before bedtime.

Take 1 teaspoon of honey before bedtime to support the production of your sleep hormone (melatonin), which gives you a deep rejuvenating beauty sleep.

4:00 - 9:00 P.M.

The skin's temperature peaks in the evening and the pores are more open, allowing the skin to sweat more. This is the perfect time for detoxifying baths, saunas and cleansing masks.

Make sure to drink water early in the evening, so you don´t dehydrate during the night.

9:00 P.M.

The skin is more histamine sensitive in the evening, which may cause itchy skin problems such as dermatitis to worsen at night. The skin's pH is more acidic in the evening, so refrain from using powerful acid treatments and peelings around this time.

4. MIDNIGHT

The production of new skin cells is at its highest around midnight. Skin renewal takes place, at its best between 9:00 p.m. – 3:00 a.m. To make the most of your beauty sleep, it is most advantageous to go to bed on the right side of midnight;)

2:00 A.M.

The skin only produces half of the amount of oil (at night), as it produces in the middle of the day, ie around 2:00 – 8:00 a.m., the skin is driest. To avoid losing moisture at night, use nourishing sera, oils and creams with plenty of moisture magnets (hyaluronic acid, honey etc) before bedtime.

Make sure to consume enough fats each day from healthy sources such as coconut, butter or ghee, avocado, fish and buckthorn. These fatty acids give hormones enough building blocks to balance themselves.

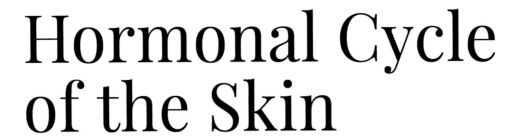

Hormonal Cycle of the Skin

The skin changes in accordance with the natural 28-day hormonal cycle

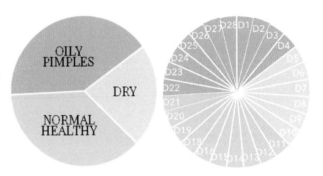

Days 5-10 /

Tendency to dry skin

The skin will typically be drier at the beginning of the cycle with a scaly tendency. Drink plenty of water, herbal tea, vegetable juices and increase the content of lecithin and healthy fats to balance the skin. We recommend using the rose quarts Gua Sha during this period.

Days 11-21 /

Normal / Optimal skin

The skin is healthiest in the days between 11-21 if you are in hormonal balance. If you have problems with PMS, you may have increased stress hormone levels that provoke the skin to produce more oil, which aggravates inflammatory skin conditions such as acne, pimples and rosacea. A relaxing self-care ritual, meditation, walks, or having fun with the family can be all it takes to increase the production of happiness hormones and thereby lowering stress hormones. Focus on an anti-inflammatory diet, rich in antioxidants,

in these days if you have an inflammatory skin problem, e.g. omega 3 from fish, turmeric, lots of vegetables and remember to spice up your food with fresh herbs. We recommend the amethyst Gua Sha during this period.

Days 22-4 /

Oily possibly with pimples

Skin is most problematic in the period from day 22-4. Skin feels greasier and there is a greater tendency to acne, dark circles under the eyes and allergic skin reactions. Increase perspiration with exercise, baths, sauna and steam baths. Clay masks are useful to clean the skin. Drink strong infusions of nettle tea daily and focus on anti-stress and blood sugar stabilizing diets. We recommend the sodalite Gua Sha during this time.

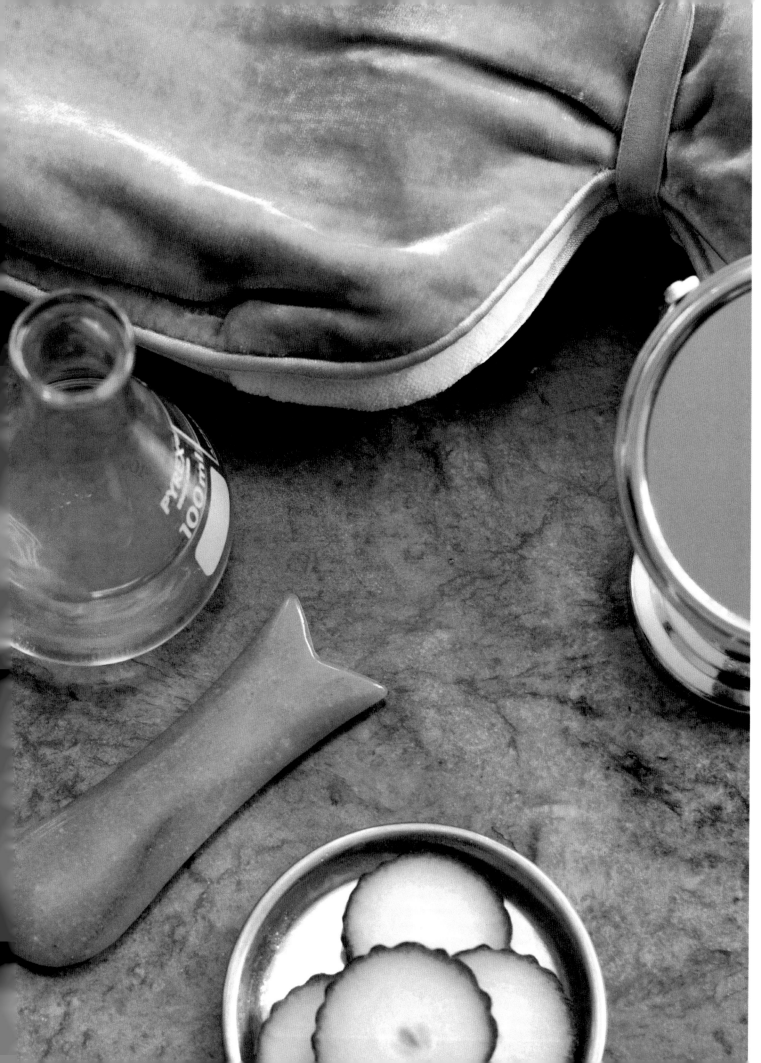

Hormonal Breakouts

If you are prone to breakouts before your period.

Hormonal outbreaks are the outbreaks of pimples that occur during the menstrual period. Use this guide to balance your skin by working with your cycle.

The 4 most important steps to regulate hormonal outbreaks:

1. Stimulate the elimination organs

When the liver is forced to work in overdrive, there is a greater risk that estrogen accumulates in the body which in turn, may cause symptoms such as breast tenderness, fluid retention, pimples and redness, especially around the chin area.

2. Ensure a healthy intestinal microbiom

As you know, an unhealthy intestinal flora contributes to systemic inflammation in the body. Inflammation is behind all skin problems. A poor digestion also lowers your ability to absorb nutrients that supply the skin's building blocks.

3. Check for nutritional deficiencies

Lack of essential vitamins, minerals and fatty acids, especially zinc, vitamin C and vitamin B contributes to pimples and acne. Make sure you get enough of these nutritional supplements from your diet.

4. Work with Your Menstrual Cycle

Your biochemistry changes with your menstrual cycle. Working with your cycle and the bodies needs in the different phases, can help you balance the skin more readily.

Balances your skin in the hormonal phases of your period. Your body goes through 4 different phases during your 28-35-day menstrual cycle:
1. Follicular phase
2. Ovulation phase
3. Luteal Phase
4. Menstrual phase

"Acne? So, remember that wound healing and healthy scarring depends, among other things, on our intake of vitamin C, vitamin E and antioxidants."

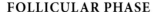

FOLLICULAR PHASE

The follicular phase starts on the first day of your cycle (i.e. the first day of your period) and ends at ovulation. In the follicular phase, hormones are at their lowest and slowly begin to rise. FSH increases to mature the egg in the ovaries. Your body needs a lot of vitality from fresh and fermented vegetables during this period.

How to support your skin and body in this phase:

- Eat 1-2 tbsp of probiotic vegetables daily with your meals. Find recipes on our blog
- Take a probiotics supplements for the night.
- Avoid wheat and dairy products at this stage to reduce inflammation.

OVULATION PHASE

In the ovulation phase, FSH and LG increase and stimulate ovulation. Estrogen and testosterone rise steadily and eventually drop again during ovulation.

How to support your skin and body in this phase:

- Drink a large glass of water with a pinch of salt and apple cider vinegar or lemon, as the first in the morning, followed by a cup of strong nettle tea to increase the elimination process in the body
- Eat 2 tbsp. freshly ground flaxseeds daily to help the excretion of used estrogen.
- Drink golden milk each evening

Goldenmilk receipe

The turmeric has anti-inflammatory benefits and helps the liver to excrete excess hormone. The other ingredients aid in absorption of the turmeric. TIP! Place a dishtowel over the lid on the blender when blending hot drinks!

Ingredients:

1 cup of 90° hot water

1 tsp honey

Blend with:

2 teaspoons turmeric

1 tsp of a good cocoa powder

1 tsp lecithin

1 tsp churned butter

1 tsp coconut oil

1/2 tsp cinnamon

½ tsp cardamom

1 pinch of black pepper

Matcha latte receipe

The turmeric has anti-inflammatory benefits and helps the liver to excrete excess hormone. The other ingredients aid in absorption of the turmeric. TIP! Place a dishtowel over the lid on the blender when blending hot drinks!

Ingredients:

1 cup of 90° hot water

1 tsp honey

Blend with:

2 teaspoons turmeric

1 tsp of a good cocoa powder

1 tsp lecithin

1 tsp churned butter

1 tsp coconut oil

1/2 tsp cinnamon

½ tsp cardamom

1 pinch of black pepper

LUTEAL PHASE

In the luteal phase, estrogen, progesterone and testosterone reach the highest and then drop to their lowest just before bleeding begins. It is during this phase that you may experience PMS if you have increased estrogen in comparison to progesterone.

How to support your skin and body in this phase:

- Replace your morning coffee with a bulletproof matcha latte made of 1 large tsp of high quality matcha (eg Japanese ippodotea.jp), 1 tsp of churned butter, 1 ttsp of coconut oil, 1 tsp of lecithin, 2 tbs collagen powder (optional) and a few drops of stevia if you prefer it sweet. This mixture will give you plenty of energy, but without stressing the nervous system. The fatty acids provide a calming effect and protect the skin from the inside. L-Theanin in the matcha makes you calm but focused.

- Have extra focus on stable blood sugar to avoid sugar cravings. That means lots of healthy fats and vegetables in all the colors of the rainbow, rich in fiber.

- Avoid facials and harsh products during this period as your skin is extra sensitive.

MENSTRUAL PHASE

Your hormones drop to their lowest at this stage and your bleeding begins.

How to support your skin and body in this phase:

- Eat foods rich in chlorophyll (the green blood of plants). Green vegetables contain a lot of minerals which are important during menstruation. The strong nettle tea infusion is rich in chlorophyll and minerals, so drink half a liter daily.

- Rub magnesium oil on the stomach and legs before bedtime to avoid cramps and menstrual discomfort.

- Place a rose quartz in your pocket. This gives a sense of peace and many claim it reduces menstrual pain.

- This is the perfect time for facials, masks, spa time and self-care.

"Freshly milled flaxseeds are one of the best sources to excrete excess "used up hormones" such as estrogen and testosterone, as the fibers bind to the hormones, so they can be secreted by the stool. This is good news if you suffer from acne or periodic pimples. Always remember to use freshly milled flaxseeds as the oil turns rancid after a few hours."

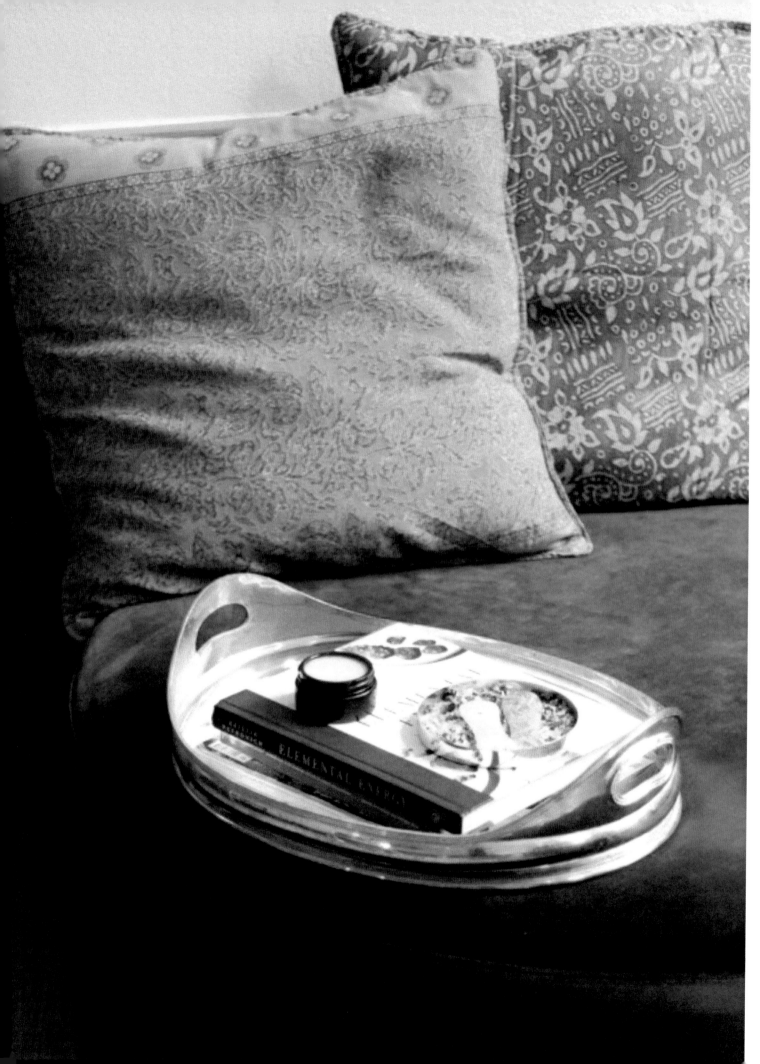

Crystal Energy

As far as we can track back in history, the human species has always been intrigued by the beauty, energy and mystery of crystals.

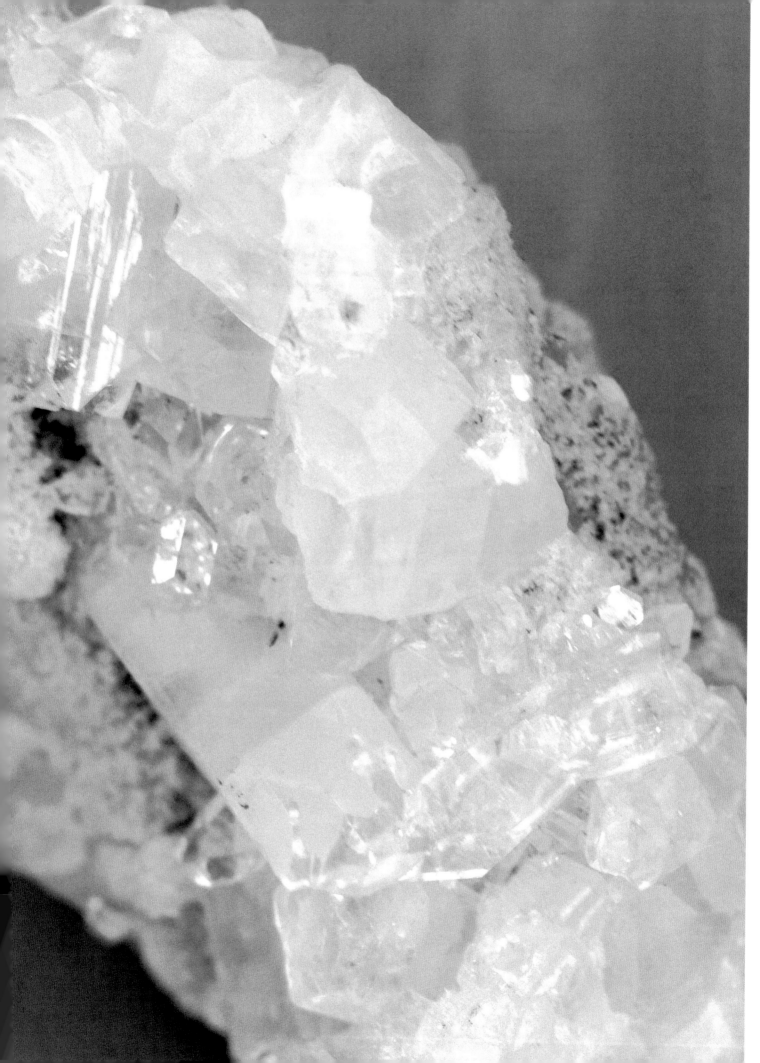

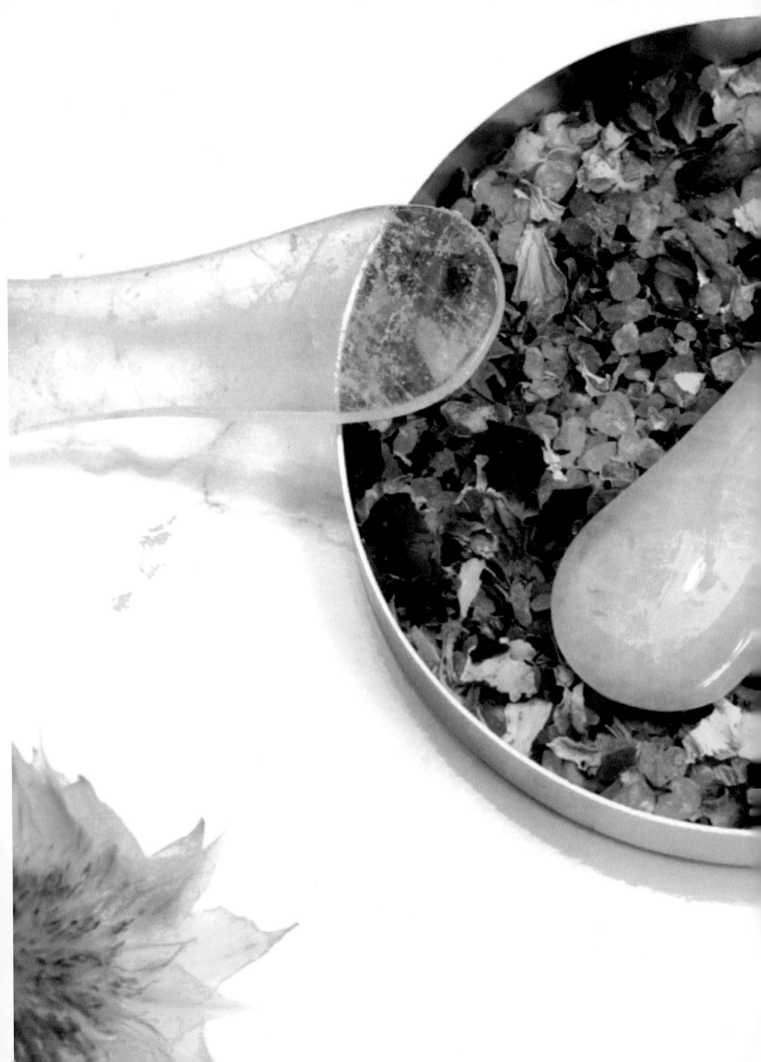

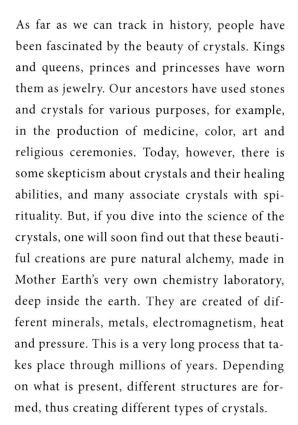

As far as we can track in history, people have been fascinated by the beauty of crystals. Kings and queens, princes and princesses have worn them as jewelry. Our ancestors have used stones and crystals for various purposes, for example, in the production of medicine, color, art and religious ceremonies. Today, however, there is some skepticism about crystals and their healing abilities, and many associate crystals with spirituality. But, if you dive into the science of the crystals, one will soon find out that these beautiful creations are pure natural alchemy, made in Mother Earth's very own chemistry laboratory, deep inside the earth. They are created of different minerals, metals, electromagnetism, heat and pressure. This is a very long process that takes place through millions of years. Depending on what is present, different structures are formed, thus creating different types of crystals.

Vibration

Each crystal releases energy and has therefore been used, through the years, to heal imbalances in the body and mind. If you think it´s difficult to understand energy, then just try to feel it in your own body. The days when you feel you have a lot of energy, are also the days when you feel your best. Those are the days where we can get up early, eat healthy, work out and achieve just about anything. They are also the days where we are most creative and able to seize new opportunities. On the other hand, there are also the days where we feel our energy is awfully low. We feel weak and beside ourselves. These are the days where we don´t achieve anything; everything is going wrong and we just wish we had stayed in bed instead. Can you recognize it? You probably also know the saying "to recharge your batteries". It´s the same as when we charge our phone.

We intuitively get the feeling that our energy is running out and we need to be recharged. Even though we don´t have a battery like our phone, there are many cultures and health systems that work with the body's energy system. For example, the Chinese work with the body's meridian system, and in India they work with the chakra system. Both systems try to balance the body's energy. The same happens when working with the vibration from crystals. Their electromagnetic field helps the body back into balance.

Healing

When we return to the old books on medical arts, we can read how crystals and precious stones were used to treat different ailments. Today, scientists have revealed that the crystal´s healing properties lie in its content of minerals. Yet, when our ancestors used crystals to relieve and cure various physical and mental illnesses, they had no scientific evidence of the crystals content. Instead, they intuitively felt what the crystals stood for/represented and what they could help with. Try, for a brief moment, to turn off your inner skeptic and just notice what you feel. Crystals are popular in skin care right now, not only because they are beautiful, but also because their subtle energy helps balance our stressed mind, which manifests itself as "tattletaling" symptoms in our skin.

We have chosen 5 different crystals and divided them up by skin type and personality. Use our descriptions, and your intuition, as a guide and choose the one that "calls out to you" and attracts you the most. There is a unique opportunity stored in every crystal that can help provide more calmness, freedom, clarity, self-love and confidence in your life.

Amethyst

CALMNESS

Amethyst is also called the stone of faith. It has a cleansing effect on the body and mind. This crystal is said to have magical powers and protects against bad energy and negative vibrations.

SKIN TYPE
Amethyst works well for normal / combination skin and is especially good for stressed / hormonal skin with periodic pimples along the jawline and on the chin.

PERSONALITY
Amethyst is for the" power woman" who needs a time-out from a busy schedule, full of commitment, and with little free time. The amethyst is for you who needs a little more calmness and gentleness in your everyday life. You can always find support; it has never been the intention that you should manage everything by yourself.

MINDSET
Amethyst gives courage, wisdom and strengthens the memory. It helps you to make the right decisions and gives self-esteem, clarity and confidence. The crystal strengthens togetherness and gives a feeling of unity, so it is easier to contain the masculine and feminine in the heart. The crystal helps you look inward and search for the real cause of your turmoil.

BODILY
Amethyst cleanses and improves blood circulation in the body. It supports our hormone system and has a destressing and calming effect. It is often used for gastro - intestinal disorders, skin disorders as well as sleep disorders. Use the amethyst to relieve headaches, neck tension and reduce wrinkles caused by tension.

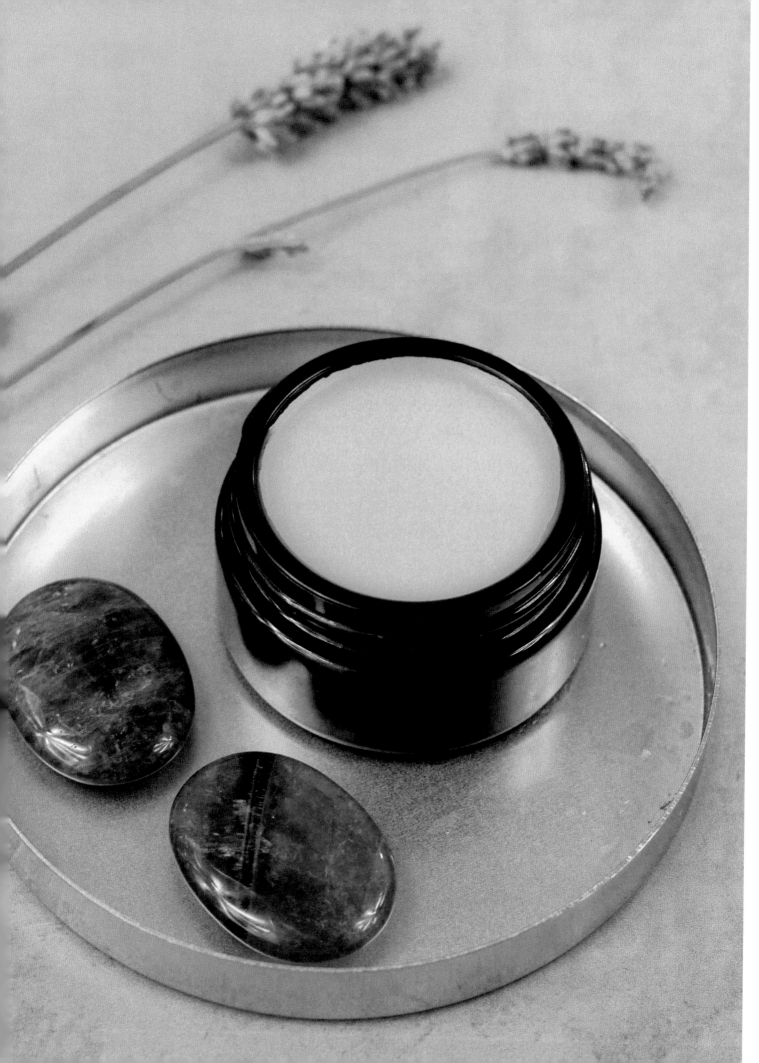

Clear Quartz

CLARITY

Clear Quartz is called the divine light or the "stone above all stones", as it contains all the colors of the rainbow. Therefore, its effect is also multifaceted. The crystal cleanses and amplifies the energy of other crystals.

SKIN TYPE
Clear quartz benefits all skin types and is a good beginner Gua Sha. It is particularly good for a dry, irritated, allergic or supersensitive skin, and if you are pregnant or breastfeeding.

PERSONALITY
Clear quartz is especially good if you need clarity and focus in a world, filled with too many choices, opportunities and requirements. Or, if you are amidst a new life transformation (eg pregnancy) and need to gather yourself, your thoughts and your energy. Gives the feeling that "someone" takes care of you.

MINDSET
Clear quartz symbolizes human growth, truth, wisdom, a sense of perspective and harmony. It gives strength, clarity and insight. It stimulates your intuitive abilities and lets you find the answer in yourself. It creates energy, unleashes the good and the positive; creates physical, mental and spiritual flow. Balances yin and yang.

BODILY
Clear quartz affects all energy centers and thus the entire body. It is a very powerful healing stone that can be used to remove illness and negative emotions. It heals everywhere in the body and is generally healing of all physical imbalances.

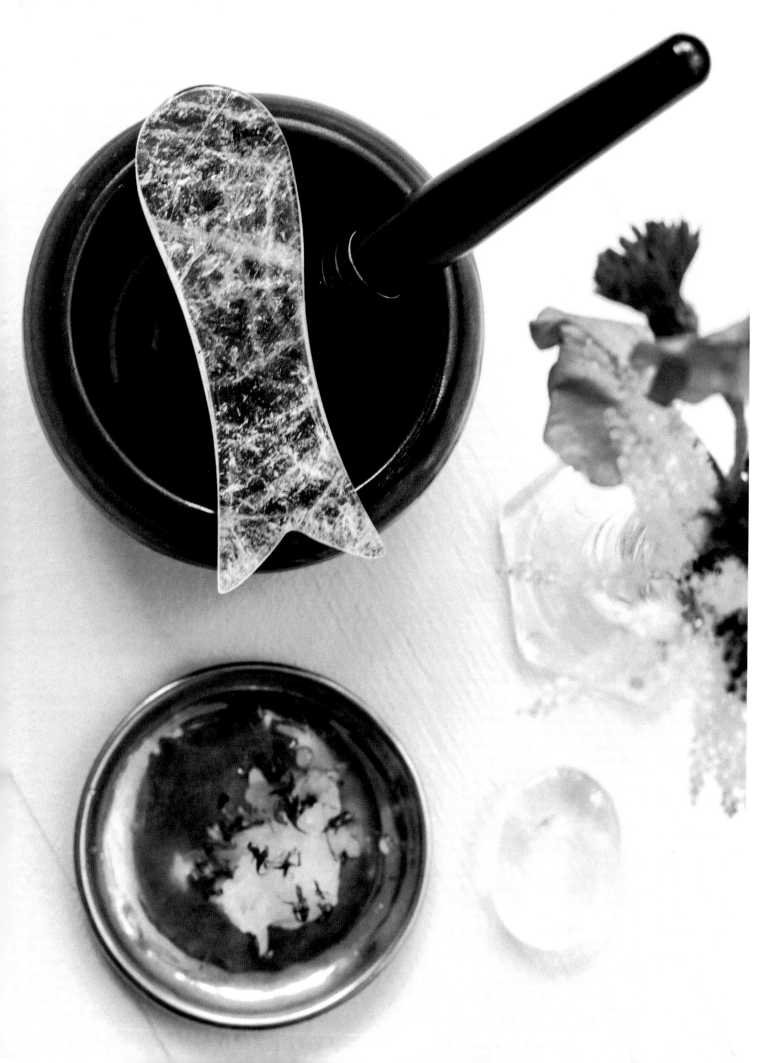

Aventurine

FREEDOM

Aventurine is called the adventurous stone. It's also known as the stone that attracts luck and feelings of abundance in all aspects of life. It represents ease, adventure and love.

SKIN TYPE
Aventurine is works well for normal or combined skin with an oily T-zone, a tendency to clogged pores and dryness on the cheeks.

PERSONALITY
Aventurine is for you who is a freedom lover and enjoys life to the fullest, but can often get stuck in duties, work overtime and a hyperactive brain. Aventurine helps you get out of your head, into the body and home to your heart, so you can breathe easy and embrace life full og adventure, love and freedom.

MINDSET
Aventurine gives you the feeling that nothing is impossible. If you feel melancholy and have lost faith in life. Or, feel lonely and cut off from the universe, then this stone is for you. It stimulates everything that is bright and positive in us. It´s good for mood swings and gives back the zest for life.

BODILY
Aventurine supports healing of skin problems and can strengthen the eyes. Aventurine works on your heart chakra.

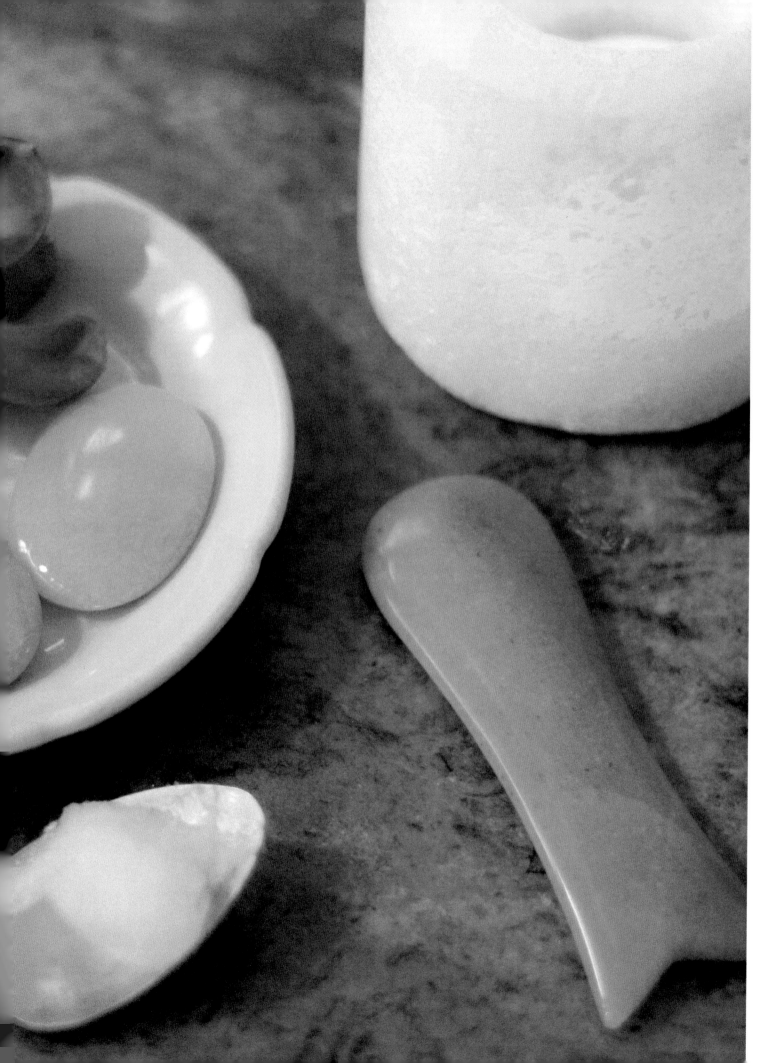

Sodalite

CONFIDENCE

Sodalite is a powerful crystal with a deep blue color. It is a stone that stands for communication and is a real initiator. It creates calmness, order, courage and a sense of perspective. Balances the masculine and feminine.

SKIN TYPE
Sodalite works well for greasy and combined skin type with a tendency to pimples and clogged pores. Additionally, it increases flow in the lymphatic system, eg with puffy eyes or fluid retention in the skin.

PERSONALITY
Sodalite is for you who wants to become better at setting boundaries. It helps you to release old fears. The sodalite is for you who seeks more confidence in yourself and the world. It helps you express your feelings, and to be a strong communicator.

MINDSET
Sodalite helps you, more than any other stone, to let go of fear and shame, and gives you the courage to change. Sodalite gives you confidence in your own assets and abilities and gives you that last push to make your vision a reality.

BODILY
Sodalite supports the throat and brow chakra (third eye chakra) so it works well on throat issues and helps to clarify why you became ill. It stimulates the lymphatic system and helps fight infections (such as pimples) as well as fluid retention and cellulite.

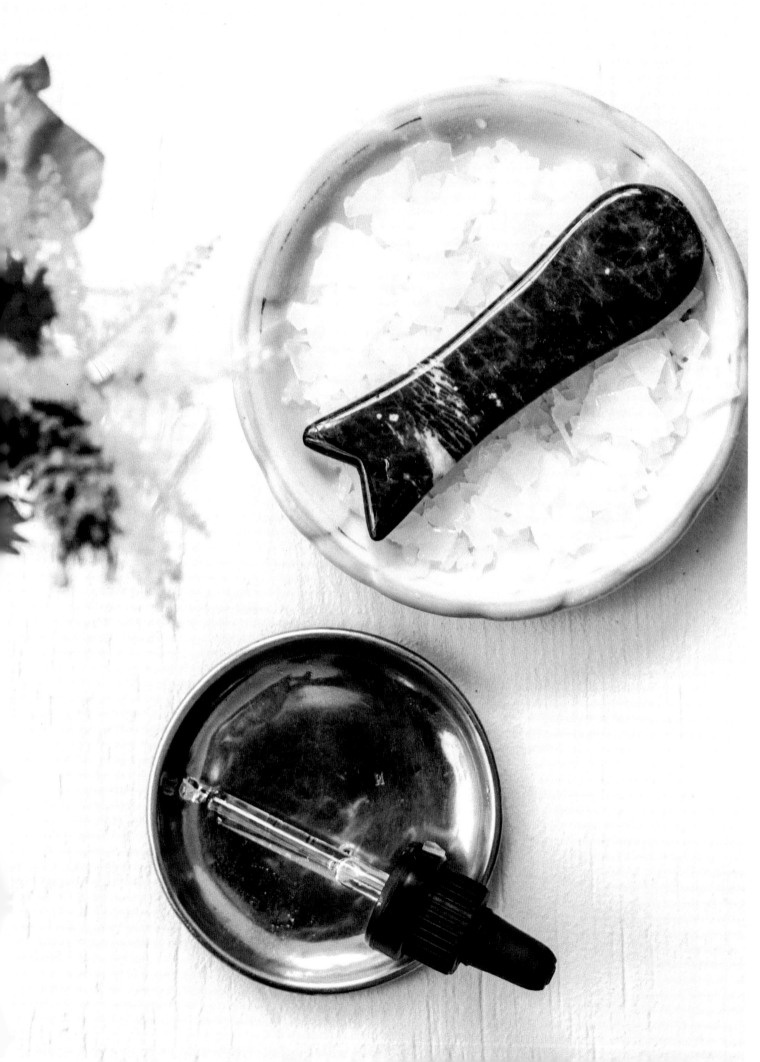

Rose Quartz

SELF-LOVE

Rose quartz is the love stone above them all. It stands for love, peace and harmony. It shields you from radiation and negative vibrations. Like the mountain crystal, it is one of the most favored stones, as it works in synergy with all other stones.

SKIN TYPE

Rose quartz works particularly well for sensitive or dry skin with a tendency to redness and wrinkles, but also a mature skin with wrinkles and loss of elasticity.

PERSONALITY

Rose quartz is for you who needs to be extra kind to yourself. For you, who needs to feel comfortable/confident again in your own skin and body. Rose quartz helps you find love for yourself and gives you a calm and peaceful mind.

MINDSET

If you are sad, anxious or insecure, rose quartz can be a good support. It gives you peace and helps you forgive. It strengthens the power of love in your life and teaches you to love yourself and the environment that surrounds you.

BODILY

Rose quartz balances the heart chakra. It radiates gentle, loving vibration and extracts negative energy from the body. Generally, it promotes healing and calmness in the whole body, thus creating balance and harmony between body and mind.

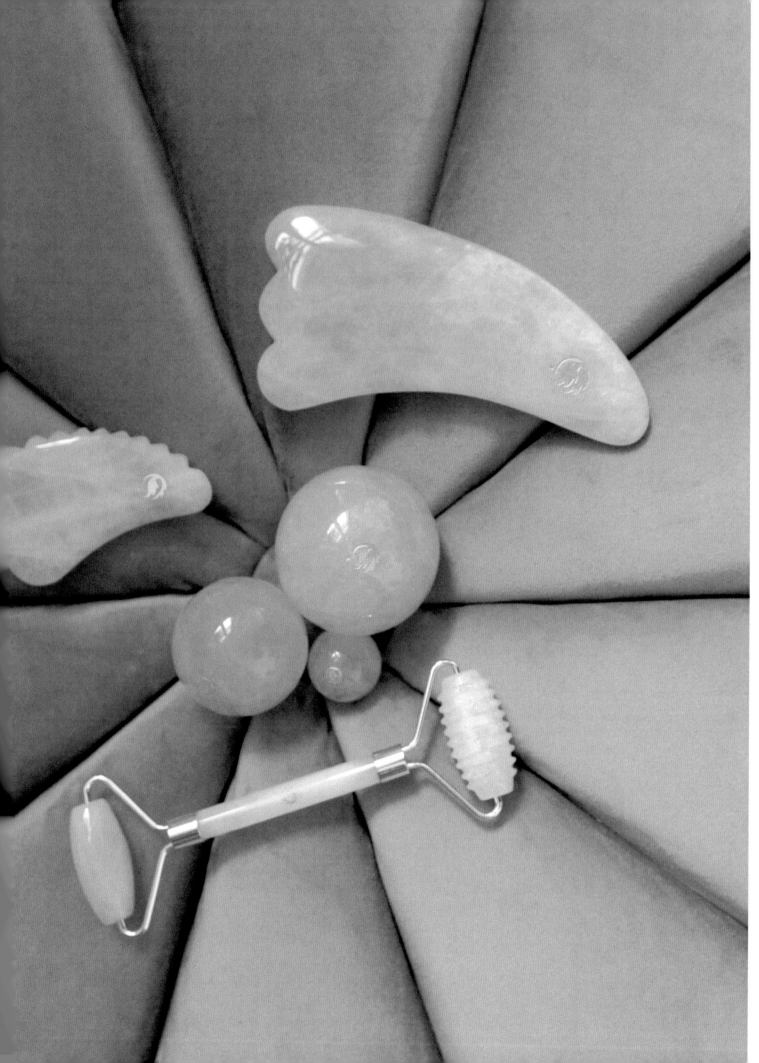

Cleanse your Crystals
Crystals carry an energy, so it's important that you remember to clean/ cleanse them.

Our Gua Sha's are unique as they are made of genuine crystals. This means that when we use them, we not only get the benefits from the massage, but we also absorb the magical properties of the individual crystal itself. Our crystals are not only chosen because they are beautiful; they are carefully selected for their healing properties, vibration and energy.

Since crystals carry an energy, it is important that they are cleaned/ cleansed optimally if you want the best out of them. Put your crystal Gua Sha in a salt water solution for 1 to 24 hours. Afterwards, rinse the Gua Sha in cold water before using it. For extra removal of bacteria, you can clean your crystal Gua Sha with rubbing alcohol, but always remember to rinse it in cold water afterwards.

Instructions
You need a bowl or a glass of water (preferably not metal) and 1 tsp of sea salt or Himalayan salt. Pour salt in tepid to hot water and place your Gua Sha in the solution after use. When you need your Gua Sha again the next evening, simply remove it from the solution and rinse it with cold water before use. Throw away the solution. Practice this after every Gua Sha massage. If you have more crystals, do not clean them in the same salt water solution.

Important: There may be some types of crystals that cannot take water; they can simply be placed on a layer of salt without water. All our crystal Gua Sha's can stand water, but do not leave them in the solution for more than 24 hours.

How to charge crystals
You can conveniently place your crystals in the window sill and thereby charge them in the sun or in the moonlight. You can also place your hand over the crystal, with a healing intention from your hand. Keep in mind, the qualities you wish from the crystal. Remember the energy always follows the intention. Hold the crystal in your left hand and use your right hand to cover it while saying the intention you want from the stone (it may be said inwardly)

Beware!
Finally, we would like to remind you that your crystal can break if you lose it on the floor. So, hold it firmly in your hand. If this mishap does occur and it breaks, you can still keep it and enjoy the benefits of the crystal. Use it as meditation stone, on the nightstand or carry it in your pocket so it can give you energy during the day.

"Our crystals are carefully selected for their skin healing properties, vibration and energy."

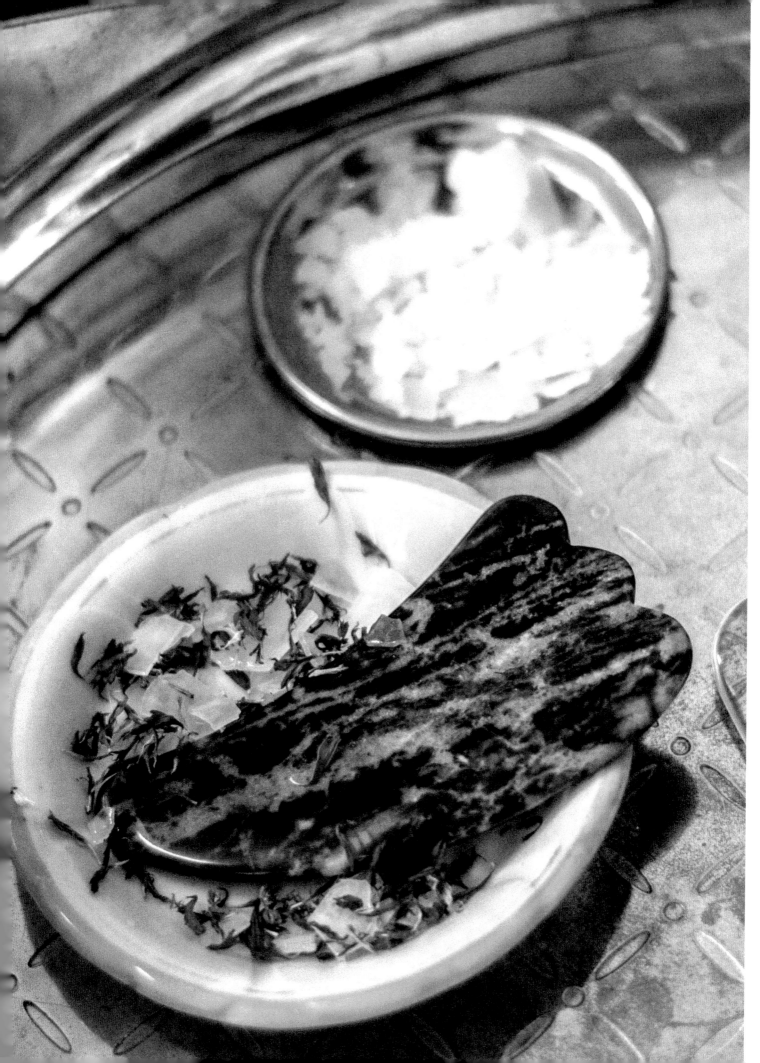

Why is Gua Sha a hit?

Today, Gua Sha is one of the most popular natural facials in Asia and is becoming a real rockstar in the beauty industry worldwide.

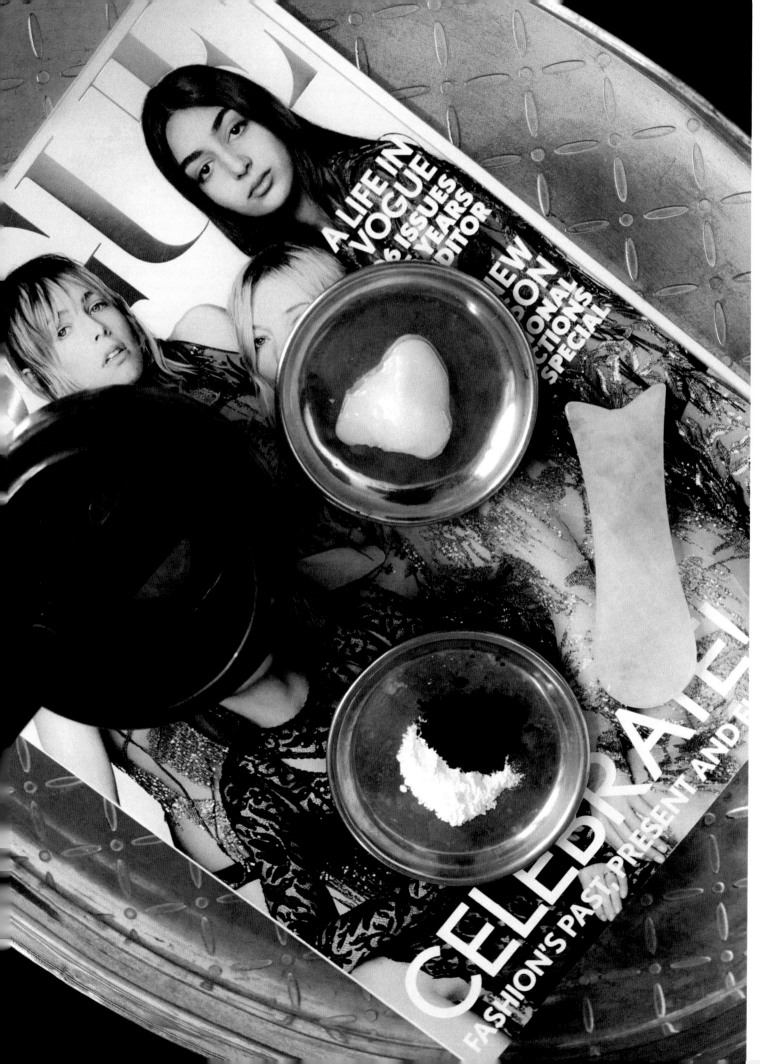

Gua Sha is a traditional Chinese healing tool that has been used for thousands of years. Today, Gua Sha is one of the most popular natural facials in Asia and is becoming a real rockstar in the beauty industry worldwide. And not without reason because the list of effects, with regular Gua Sha massage, makes it really worth a try.

Improves blood circulation

- Creates a youthful glow in the skin
- Activates cells to restore skin elasticity
- Reduces wrinkles
- Reduces pores
- Promotes skin smoothness
- Removes / reduces dark circles and bags under the eyes
- Improves muscle tone and lifts facial skin
- Provides a more even skin tone
- Removes stagnant lymphatic fluid and toxins
- Provides a healthy and younger appearance

Chinese folk medicine

Gua Sha is an ancient healing technique, originating from China. It is an essential part of traditional Chinese medicine, used as folk medicine in many Chinese homes. It´s origin dates back thousands of years and involves scraping the skin to eliminate toxins, waste products, tension and pain.

Gua means "to scrape" and Sha means "red spots / redness". It is a highly effective treatment that provides immediate benefits. The tools used to scrape with, are special Gua Sha tools. In our treatments, we have chosen to combine Gua Sha with crystal healing. Therefore, our Gua Sha tools are made in crystal stone.

The Gua Sha Treatment

The principle behind the Gua Sha technique is to repeatedly scrape, on a lubricated skin area, with a Gua Sha tool. One scrapes in a certain direction, eg from acupuncture points, meridian pathways and lymphatic pathways.

In our Gua Sha facials, we remove tension, stagnant energy and toxins and drain them to our lymphatic system. Gua Sha works by promoting the vital energy "Qi", stimulates blood circulation and removes stagnant blood and fluid retention.

For example, we can compare it to a highway. Even if we drive in a brand new sportscar, rather than an old slow car, we can´t get there faster if there is a traffic jam. The same applies if there is no flow in our energy, blood and lymphatic system. When an area is treated by repeated "scraping/ rubbing", a vacuum occurs which causes toxic fluid to be drawn to the skin from the underlying tissue of the body.

This toxic fluid is seen as "Sha" or the red spots that appear on the skin after treatment. The darker the spots are, the more old and stagnant the blood has been in that area. When we work on the face, we do not press as hard because the skin is more sensitive, so the redness disappears quickly. The expulsion of Sha literally means to draw the "stagnation" from the inside to the surface and away from the body.

To be exact, we do not work in such depth when we work on the face. The Chinese call it "Shu" instead of "Sha". It is a lighter red color, not like the dark red, purple and blue color that can be seen on the body.

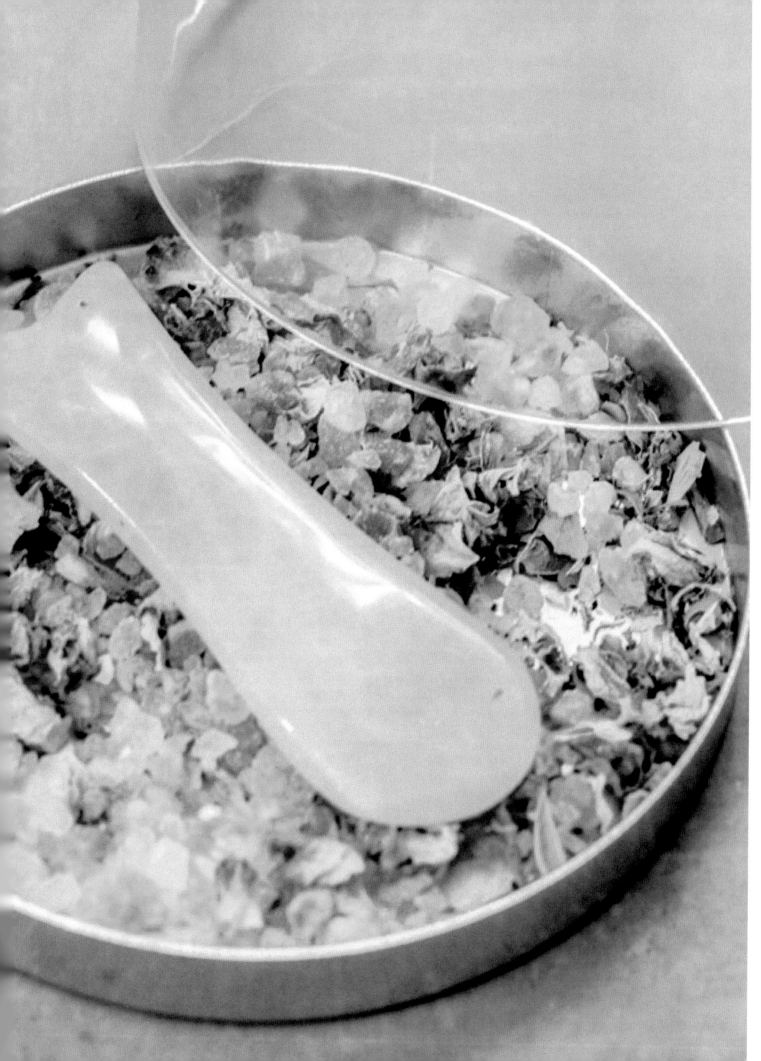

Contraindications

Gua Sha massage is not ideal if you have the following:

• Sunburned skin
• candida fungus skin infection
• Inflamed skin
• Wounds
• Damaged skin
• Skin cancer
• Illness
• Swollen lymph nodes
• Fever

NB: If you are in doubt, always ask your doctor. Be aware if you are taking medication, especially if it is blood thinning. If you have any type of blood disorders or have extra sensitive skin due to illness and medicine, always remember to consult your doctor first.

What You Need for Your Gua Sha Massage

All you need is a Gua Sha tool and an oil / balm. We always use a facebalm that suits our skin type (we use a bodybalm for the body) because creams and serums are often absorbed too quickly into the skin. To avoid damaging the skin, it is important that you have a product on the skin before rubbing with your Gua Sha tool. Your Gua Sha Facial is also perfect in aiding the absorption of your products, making your skin look better.

Our Crystal Gua Sha Massage

In our DIY Facials we have chosen to combine traditional Gua Sha techniques with lymphatic drainage, acupressure, facial zone therapy, connective tissue massage, respiratory therapy, crystal healing, aromatherapy and classic lifting and relaxation techniques.

Our goal has been to make an easy and effective self-treatment technique that can be safely performed at home. The concept behind this, is that you can take care of the beauty and health of your skin in a 100% natural, non- invasive and sustainable manner.

How the treatment works

Acupressure: Through our meridian system, we can tap into our life energy, flowing like our blood flows into our arteries and veins. This life energy is extremely important to keep in balance as it regulates our health, wellbeing and appearance. This is no new science; this system is more than 5000 years old and has been used, by the Chinese, for ages.

Breathing exercises and acupressure relax muscle tension and balance the vital energy of the body. Your vitality or your life energy flows between the body's meridians. Acupuncture points are locations where you can tap into that energy.

When the pressure accumulates around one point, it blocks the energy from flowing optimally. This creates an excess of energy in an area of the face and a deficiency in another area. The pressure is gathered around the acupuncture points and eventually blocks the circulation, which consequently results in a wrinkle. The massage technique naturally pushes and stretches the nerves and muscles, while the acupuncture points release tension, so the energy can flow freely. These blockages can be avoided by performing the massage regularly. Gua Sha tones the face and stimulates the body's natural self-healing abilities.

Our meridian pathways are also connected to our organs. If we want healthy skin, it´s imperative that our organs function sufficiently. When your organs are working overtime, all nutrition will go to them. We can compare our skin with a leaf. If the root does not nourish the leaf, it withers and eventually, the leaf falls off. Similarly, the skin needs our organs to function optimally, so we can provide proper nourishment to the skin and thereby prevent the skin from withering.

To maintain a beautiful and healthy face, it is vital that our organ system is in balance. For example. our heart cannot function optimally without our kidneys as the heart produces heat (the fire element) and the kidneys are cooling (the water element). If the imbalance becomes too great and the entire system becomes overheated, it may appear on the skin as acne, rosacea and broken capillaries. On the other hand, if the system becomes too cold, it may appear as puffiness of the face, sagging skin and pigmentation.

The Connective Tissue
The connective tissue is a substance that lies between the skin and the muscles. Over time, the connective tissue becomes weak and releases itself from the muscles. This results in wrinkles and saggy skin. With the right techniques, we can strengthen the connection between our skin and muscles. The circulation is increased, resulting in a better facial skin tone.

The Lymphatic System
Lymphatic drainage is an important part of our Crystal Gua Sha treatments. In almost all our facials, and on the body, we work with the drainage of lymphatic fluid to the lymph nodes.

During absorption of nutrients from the blood capillaries to the body, excess fluid is released into the body´s tissue. This is called lymph; in Latin, Lympha means "clear water". Lymphatic fluid is a clear liquid, which consists of a variety of waste products from cells in the body's tissues. It can also contain foreign microorganisms or particles such as bacteria, viruses, etc. Lymphatic capillaries are thin vessels that absorb the fluid. Each lymphatic capillary carries lymph into a lymphatic vessel, which in turn connects to a lymph node. When the lymphatic fluid reaches the lymph nodes, it is cleansed and returned to the venous circulation. It is safe to say that our lymph nodes are the body´s detoxification plant. When working with lymphatic drainage, we always work in the direction of the lymphatic pathways. If the lymphatic system is damaged or its function somehow impaired, the fluid will accumulate in the skin. This can result in a lymphedema which causes swelling, pain and increased risk of infection. The lymph´s primary task is to remove the excess fluid from the skin and rid the body of foreign microorganisms and toxins. With the help of lymphatic drainage, we can stimulate the lymphatic circulation and thus remove lymphatic edema in the skin. By stimulating the lymph, we can also treat many different skin conditions such as pimples, cellulite and redness. We have about 900 lymph nodes in the body, 200 of which are in the neck. Lymph nodes are bean-shaped structures, varying in size, from a few mm to about 2 cm.

"By stimulating the lymph. we can treat many different skin conditions such as pimples. cellulite and redness."

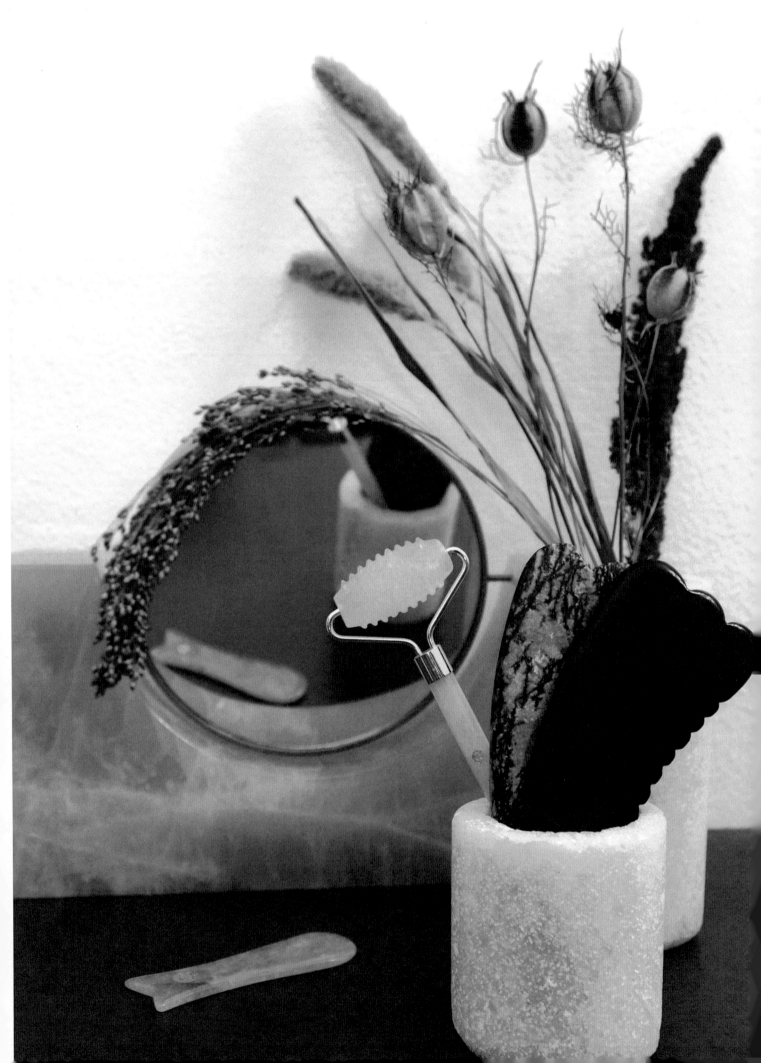

Breathing is another important part of our Gua Sha massage which is usually not something we tend to think about in our daily lives. Our body is so intelligent that it breathes for us, all by itself, to keep us alive. Our breath is the most important thing we have. If we stop breathing, we die. It's plain and simple. Breathing is something that happens automatically in our body and is the most fundamental tool we have. We can actually optimize it by being conscious of using our breath optimally. It may seem ironic that we must learn to breathe correctly, but why only use your breath to keep you alive. Why not take advantage of your natural superpower and move on to a world where you become more present in your body, more conscious and awake. A natural, healthy breath is a free way to fill the body with energy and vitality.

How to breathe correctly

Think of the way a baby breathes and notice the way their stomach rises and falls, each time they take a breath., Make sure you breathe all the way down to your abdomen. That way, you obtain optimal oxygen absorption and you reduce your stress levels which in turn, will give you an energy surplus on your health and beauty account.

How it Works

Your breath is only taking place in the present, so when you begin to breathe consciously, in a mindful manner, you cannot avoid being aware of the present moment. If you have a flow of negative thoughts and worry too much about the future and the past, your breathing can help to bring you back to the present and draw you away from your thoughts. Thus, helping you to connect on a spiritual level. In yoga, it is said that breathing helps regulate and channel the flow of vitality through the subtle body.

Because your breath is immaterial, it also connects us with the intangible and unknown in the universe. We feel more connected when we focus on our breath. Practicing breathing exercises through Pranayama techniques, can be beneficial to your health, vitality and consciousness; especially in the busy lives we lead where we lack time for relaxation and well-being. Here your magic breath is a complimentary way to calm your autonomic nervous system and balance your body.

In all our Gua Sha treatments, we recommend that you focus on your breath. This will help you to ease tension, stagnant energy and unresolved feelings. When we take long deep breaths, we use the full capacity of our lungs by utilizing the 3 chambers of the lungs:

- Abdominal (lower part)
- The breast (the middle part)
- Clavicular (the upper part)

Long deep breathing starts with filling the abdominal cavity, expanding the chest and then lifting the upper ribs and collar bone. Upon exhalation the exact opposite occurs; first the upper part decreases, then the middle part, and eventually the abdominal cavity is pulled in and up as the navel point is retracted towards the spine.

In the practical part of the book, we show you how to do our DIY Gua Sha Facials. Don´t hesitate to send us an email if you have any questions, or if you are in doubt whether you are practicing it right. Remember, we are here to help you, so you can feel the amazing results of the Gua Sha massage and the Slow Beauty lifestyle. We would also really appreciate your feedback and personal experiences with the Gua Sha massage.

DIY Skincare

Everything around us is energy and everything has its own vibration, including your skincare, if you practice it with love, care and presence.

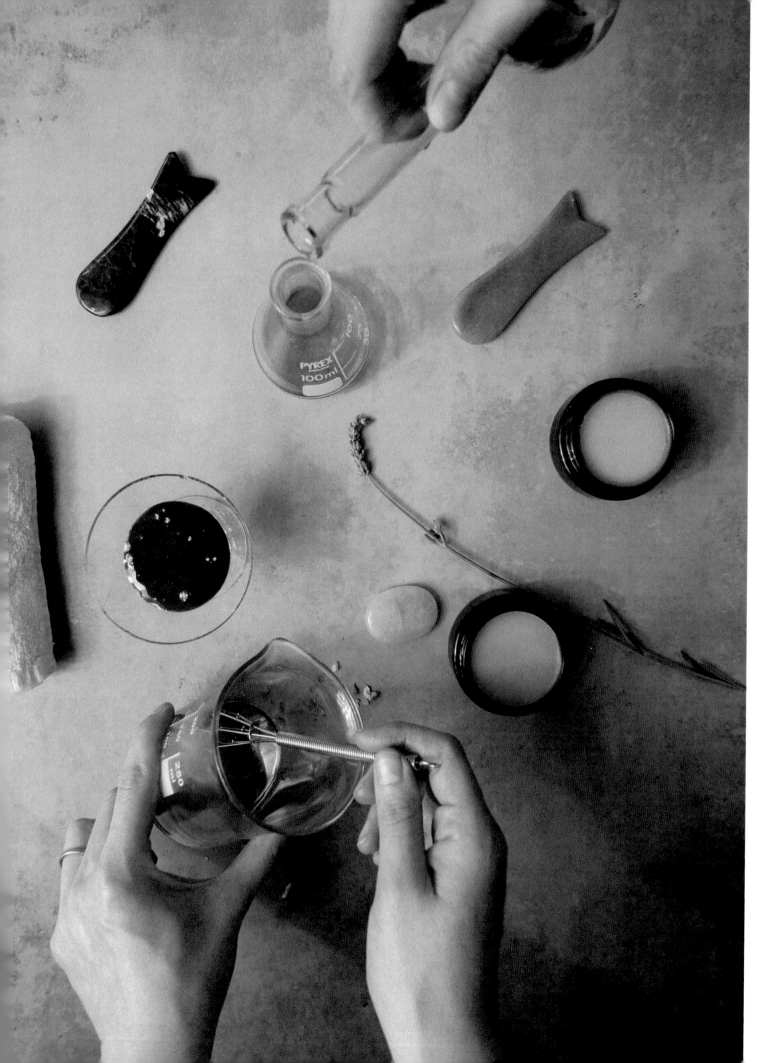

Creating Beauty through the Science of Scent

The reasons why you will love using aromatherapy in your skin care

Scents and aromatic plants have always been part of the beauty care of all cultures.

Certain scents are associated with a particular mood or feeling. We use this association deliberately in aromatherapy. For example, with winter depression, we use scents that remind us of a particular season, to balance our inner condition, through the sense of smell; directly connected to the brain's center for memories and feelings. The smell of mint, for example, is associated with something fresh, and something fresh relates to a fresh summer day, feeling clean, or a mouthwatering beverage on the beach, cocktails, etc.

In aromatherapy, we only use genuine essential oils, which are concentrated extracts from powerful healing compounds in plants. The oils work intensely on skin, body and mind; at the same time. In fact, essential oils are some of the only active skin care ingredients that have proven to be in all layers of the skin and in the bloodstream. They can do this in less than an hour. When you take a deep breath and smell the essential oil, it will be in your bloodstream almost instantly.

Holistic aromatherapy is therefore more than just a scent. Holistic aromatherapy is a gentle and non-invasive therapy that increases the sense of well-being and balance. It strengthens the immune system, increases resilience, lowers stress and gently dissolves psychosomatic roots/

energy (such as many skin conditions). The holistic aromatherapy supports your body's own healing process, rather than symptomatic treatment of a specific symptom or disease.

Most importantly, it feels delightful and self-loving to nourish yourself with a "scent moment" that you have deliberately chosen to meet exactly what you need. The fragrance follows you all day and reminds you of your personal intention for yourself.

The essential oils, used in our facebalm recipes, have been carefully selected not only to suit skin type, but also to treat emotional stressors behind the various skin problems. With intelligent aromatherapy compositions, we have created small scent universes that bring you closer to yourself. In addition to using aromatherapy facebalms, we always have an aromatherapy roll-on in the bag for a fast-anti-stress fix. You will also receive the recipes for these rescue roll-ons´.

"With intelligent aromatherapy compositions, we have created small scent universes that bring you closer to yourself."

How do you know which fragrance to choose? Use our descriptions of the various essential oils and take note of the ones you feel apply to you. Go to a good health food store and smell the ones you have noted, then choose the ones you love the most. Your nose is the best intuitive guide.

Are you fortunate enough to go to Paris, then go to one of our favorite shops Aroma Zone or Florame. They have a huge selection of oils of good quality. Or come in to one of our many workshops and "smell away." Alternatively, you can choose one of our recipes that suits your skin the best.

CLARY SAGE

Clary Sage is one of the "woman oils" that we love to use on our skin to prevent hormonal break-outs. It has a cleansing effect on the skin, seems uplifting and balances the mood. The fragrance is spring-like, light and feminine, but with an edge of mystery and wildness that we love. You can find it in our violet and green balm.

LAVENDER

Lavender oil is one of the most skin-healing and soothing essential oils we have. Lavender has a calming floral scent with fresh herbal notes. We love to use lavender in our cleansing oil in the evening, and to dab a few drops on our pillow for extra deep beauty sleep.

GREEN MANDARIN

Green Mandarin is a fresh and more acidic version of the soothing Mandarin, which can boost any mixture of essential oils. We use Mandarin because of its pore cleansing properties. Be careful not to use large amounts of citrus oils in the daytime as they can interact with the sun in a negative way. In our recipes, we use just the right amount, so you can safely use them. However, we recommend that you perform your Gua Sha massage in the evening. That way, the oils have already been absorbed in the bloodstream before the next morning.

LINDEN FLOWER

Linden flower is spring freshness in drops; used in aromatherapy to give a sense of cheerful ease, reawakened with new energy and courage. In all our aromatherapy workshops, linden flower has been the absolute favorite because of its light floral breezy scent.

VIOLA/ VIOLET LEAF ABSOLUTE

Viola leaves have an intense fragrance of fresh green leaves with notes of violets and rain, when diluted in a facebalm. In aromatherapy, the green fragrances are applied to give a feeling of "breathing deeply", like going for a long walk in the woods to dissolve stress, anxiety and heavy thoughts. We love viola in skincare because of its detoxifying, skin-renewing and tightening properties.

TUBEROSE

Tuberose is femme fatale in a bottle, but in the good way. Tuberose is called the queen of the night, as it is used in aromatherapy for those in search of true love. The sweet powdery exotic fragrance goes straight to the heart. It is extremely calming on the nervous system and creates / brings out feelings of joy and peace.

VETIVER

Vetiver is the fragrance of grounding and connects you energetically to the earth. If you spend most of your time dealing with things in your head, vetiver is the oil for you! It takes you straight back to your body, so you can relax. The scent reminds us of a wet earthy forest after a rainfall and is used in aromatherapy to relieve stress, anxiety, mood swings, mental and emotional hyperactivity. We use it in skin care because of its skin-calming, protective and rejuvenating properties. It is suitable for stressed and inflamed skin conditions. We call it "Zen for the skin."

ROSE

The Rose fragrance has an intense scent of summery rose petals with a hint of green, spicy notes. Rose is used in aromatherapy to heal sorrow and bereavement. It also helps during PMS and has an uplifting effect on the mood. We use rose in skin care for its regenerating, healing and antibacterial properties for sensitive skin, mature skin and skin with pimples and acne. Rose stimulates the microcirculation of the skin and is therefore used for broken capillaries and redness.

HELICHRYSUM

Helichrysum has a spicy floral scent with a hint of tea and is extremely relaxing. Helichrysum is a skin favorite as it is healing, renewing, draining and bactericidal. Therefore, it can be used for all skin concerns such as bruising, swelling, acne, redness, broken capillaries, scars and wrinkles.

COCOA ABSOLUTE

Cocoa smells of chocolate and provides a soft and mellow base for aromatherapy mixtures. Cocoa contains skin-protective antioxidants, and we use it to prevent premature skin aging.
Ylang ylang
Ylangs fragrance is exotic and floral with notes of jasmine and camphor. The aroma is complex, heavy and feminine and is used in aromatherapy to strengthen the mind-body connection. We use Ylang Ylang in skin care to treat combination skin with a tendency to pimples as it balances the sebum production and has antibacterial benefits.

BLUE TANSY

Blue tansy is probably the most hyped essential oil currently, and for good reason. Its beneficial skin properties are calming and anti-inflammatory, and suit sensitive, dry, ruddy and oily skin. The scent is wild and certainly not one, you have the smelled before. It is deep, herbal, sweet and complex, and a little goes a long way in your facebalm. Did we mention that it colors your facebalm the most beautiful light blue color? It is the anti-inflammatory substance, Azulene, which makes the color. Blue tansy is used in aromatherapy to soothe frustration, impatience and irritation (for all us control freaks) and helps us let go of what we can´t control anyway

YUZU

Yuzu is a fresh citrus fruit; very popular in Japan. The light scent takes you out into the sunshine with fresh air and clears your head. We use it in skin care for its pore cleansing effect. In aromatherapy, Yuzu is used to help combat fatigue and emotional stress.

Yuzu is most often distilled; not extracted by high pressure which means it does not contain phototoxic substances like cold pressed citrus oils often do.

FRANKINCENSE

Frankincense is pure meditation for your mind and your skin. Frankincense is one of the oldest aromatic plants and has been used in religious ceremonies for thousands of years, due to its meditative and cleansing scent. Frankincense smells fresh and mysterious with notes of wood, camphor and flowers. The scent gives a sense of elevation and a feeling of space to be just as you are. Frankincense is popular in skin care and is the significant ingredient in many of Neal's Yard's products. We use frankincense in skin care for its skin healing, regenerating, scar healing and anti-wrinkle properties. It is also used to combat sun damage, pigmentation and redness after acne.

BLUE CYPRESS

Blue cypress has a scent of forest and wood and is used in aromatherapy to clear the mind. Relieve stress and give a "breath of fresh air" during stressful periods. We use cypress in skin care because of it stimulates skin renewal, strengthens blood vessels, stimulates microcirculation and detoxifies the skin. Therefore, it is the supporting element of our body detox balm.

NEROLI

Nerolis fragrance is that of citrus flowers and southern summer heat. Neroli is used in aromatherapy to give a sense of deep peace, confidence and protection. We call it the "protection pupa" as it gives a sense of entering a pupa that shields you from the world's stressful environment. We love to use neroli to treat delicate and reactive skin that especially responds to stress and emotional conditions. Neroli is regenerating and soothing on the skin.

GRAPEFRUIT

The fragrance of the grapefruit is tangy with a floral note which gives it an interesting edge. Grapefruit is used in aromatherapy to awaken and "rebuild" yourself after demanding periods. We use grapefruit in our detox body balm for its cleansing, draining and firming properties.

GINGER LILY + VETIVER

Ginger lily + vetiver is a special combination of the honey-blossoming, white butterfly ginger and the deep earthy vetiver. The result is a deeply grounded, but elevating scent that completely relaxes the nervous system. You cannot help closing your eyes and taking a deep breath when you smell it. We think the scent takes us, mentally, on an adventure to a quiet forest lake and the exotic jungle. We use it in skincare to treat stressed skin that needs rest and rejuvenation.

Bestseller Facebalms

The solid facial oils are the perfect complement to your Gua Sha facial.

We always use a facebalm that suits our skin type when we perform Gua Sha Facials. It is important that you have a product, with the right texture for your skin, before rubbing with your Gua Sha tool so you don´t damage the skin. The reason why facebalms are such a hit, lies in their firm consistency which consists of a special composition of fatty acids that simultaneously protects and repairs the skin barrier, without leaving the skin greasy or with clogged pores.

Facebalms are compact facial oils with an extra protection factor, which derives from skin-loving butters from kokum and sheabutter. Butters are solid fatty acids that protect the skin from moisture loss and repair the skins barrier.

When the butters are mixed with the moisture boosting squalane, the product will have the most delightful texture that is solid in the jar but will melt upon contact with the skin. The facebalms are only made of squalane, essential oils and butters which means they are quickly absorbed without leaving a greasy residue on the skin.

Use a facebalm as a Gua Sha base or as a cream morning and evening. Your skin will feel silky, protected and moisturized throughout the day.

HOW TO MAKE THE PERFECT FACEBALM

STEP 1
Choose the right recipe for your skin type and follow these simple steps to make the perfect facebalm.

STEP 2
Weigh your butters in a glass measuring cup or bowl and heat in an electronic chocolate melter or melt over a water bath at low heat until completely melted.

STEP 3
In another measuring cup or bowl, weigh squalane, rosemary CO2 extract, possibly castor oil / hemp oil / color, if stated in your recipe. Blend well. When your butters are melted, mix them with this oil mixture and stir well.

STEP 4
Now add the essential oils and stir thoroughly. If your recipe requires the azulene or alkane extract (color), then add until desired color is achieved. When your facebalm is solid, the color will get a bit brighter.

STEP 5
Make a water bath in a small bowl with ice cubes. Place the cup with the balm mixture in, and hold it firmly, so it doesn´t tip. Stir until the mixture becomes thick and you can draw visible lines in it with a whisk. The color will go from transparent to milky and the texture will get thicker. Pour it onto your 50 ml glass jar before it gets too thick to pour. This cooling process ensures a smooth and delightful texture. If you skip this step, your balm will be gritty. Place the jar in the refrigerator for 30 minutes and it´s ready for use. Your balm can last for 9 months with regular storage. Remember to use a spatula, and not your fingers, when removing it from the jar.

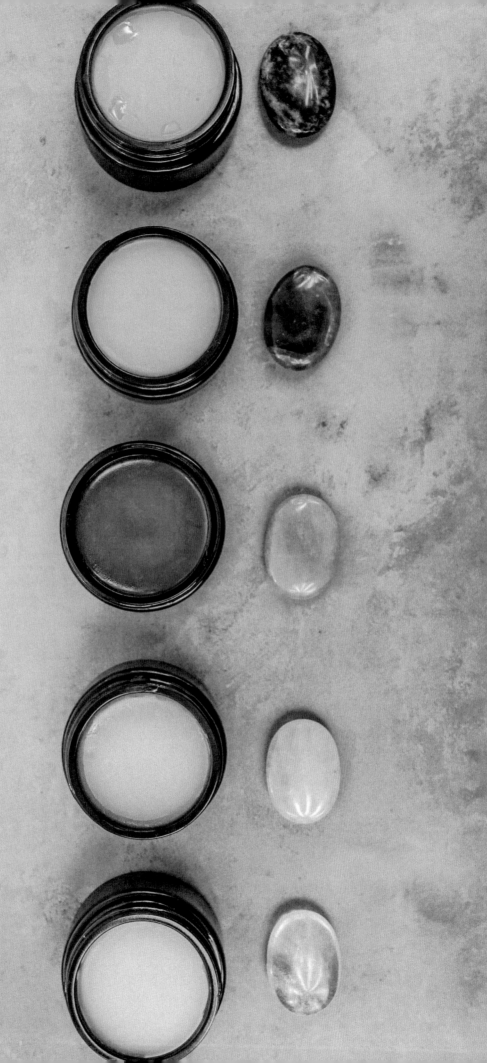

Calmness

Calmness works especially well on the stressed/ hormonal skin type, which needs a time-out from a hectic lifestyle with too many obligations and not enough time for relaxation. You don´t have to do everything yourself; you can always find support.

SKIN TYPE

Our Calmness Balm contains a relaxing, mildly cleansing and balancing aromatherapeutic blend of lavender, clary sage, vetiver, linden flower, viola, tuberose and green mandarin. These ingredients optimize the normal skin type and eliminate periodic breakouts

INGREDIENTS

15g	kokum butter
15g	sheabutter
15g	squalane
5g	Ricinus oil or castor oil
5	drops of rosemary CO2 extract
2	drops of lavender
1	drop of vetiver
1	drop of viola
2	drops of tuberose
3	drops of linden flower
3	drops of clary sage
3	drops of green mandarin

SUPPLIES NEEDED

- Digital scale, weighing down to 1 gram

- 2 small glass measuring cups or bowls or stainless-steel bowls (available in our webshop)

- A chocolate melter or just a bowl for a water bath

- 1 mixing utensil or a small whisk

- 1 tea filter

- 1 50ml jar in dark glass

- 1 tbsp alkanet root

- approx. 5 drops of azulene extract

PROCEDURE

Start by extracting 1 tbsp. alkanet root in approx. 30 ml of squalane oil. Leave it in a warm water bath for about an hour. Strain the alkanet root from the oil by pouring it through a tea filter, so you have a pure red oil left over. Mix the red oil with approx. 5 drops of azulene extract, or as much as it requires, to turn the mixture purple. Follow the instructions from the "Bestseller Facebalms" section. Page 66.

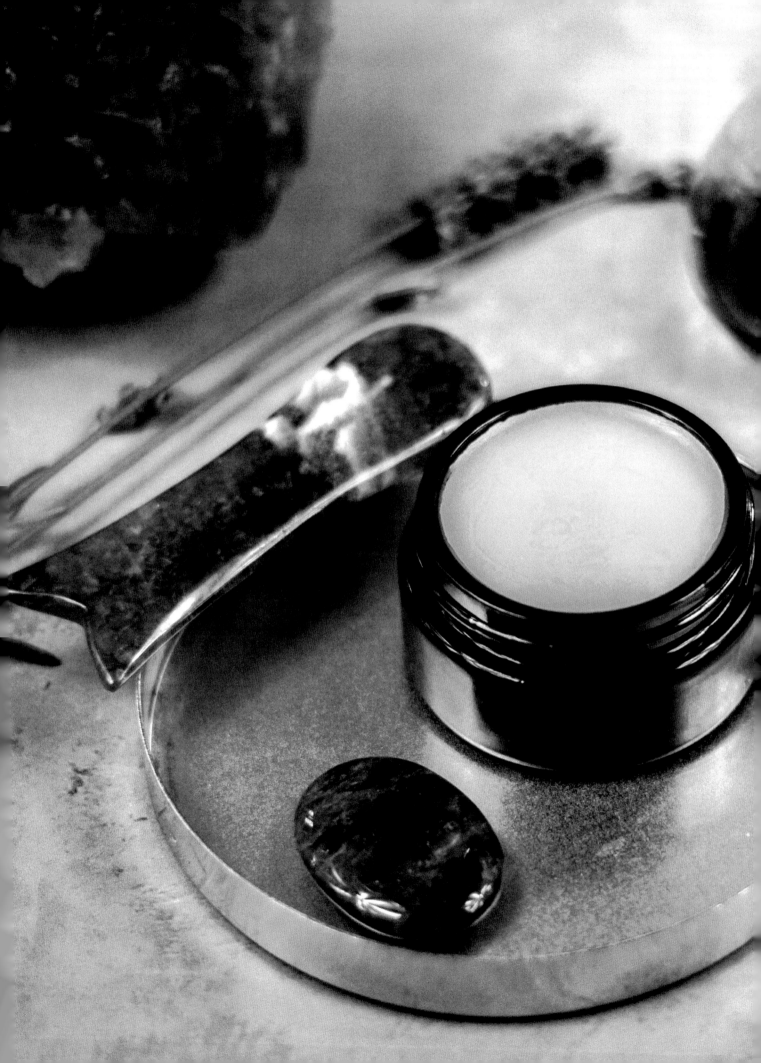

Self-Love

Self-love is especially good for the sensitive, dry and / or mature skin. It also applies to you who wants to be kind to yourself, with a need to feel confident and comfortable again in your own skin and body. You are enough.

SKIN TYPE

Our Self-Love Balm contains a calming, antioxidant rich, anti-inflammatory and healing aromatherapeutic blend of rose, cocoa, lavender, helichrysum and ylang ylang. These ingredients repair the skin barrier, reduce fine lines and wrinkles, and relieve redness and irritation.

INGREDIENTS

15g	kokum butter
15g	sheabutter
20g	squalane
5	drops of rosemary CO2 extract
1	tbsp alkanet root
4	drops of lavender
2	drops of ylang ylang
1	drop of helichrysum
3	drops of cocoa absolute
2	drops of rose

SUPPLIES NEEDED

- Digital scale, weighing down to 1 gram

- 2 small glass measuring cups or bowls or stainless-steel bowls (available in our webshop)

- A chocolate melter or just a bowl for a water bath

- 1 mixing utensil or a small whisk

- 1 tea filter

- 1 50ml jar in dark glass

PROCEDURE

Start by extracting 1 tbsp. alkanet root in approx. 30 ml of squalene oil. Leave it in a warm water bath for about an hour. Strain the alkanet root from the oil by pouring it through a tea filter, so you have a pure red oil left over. Follow the instructions from the "Bestseller Facebalms" section. Page 66.

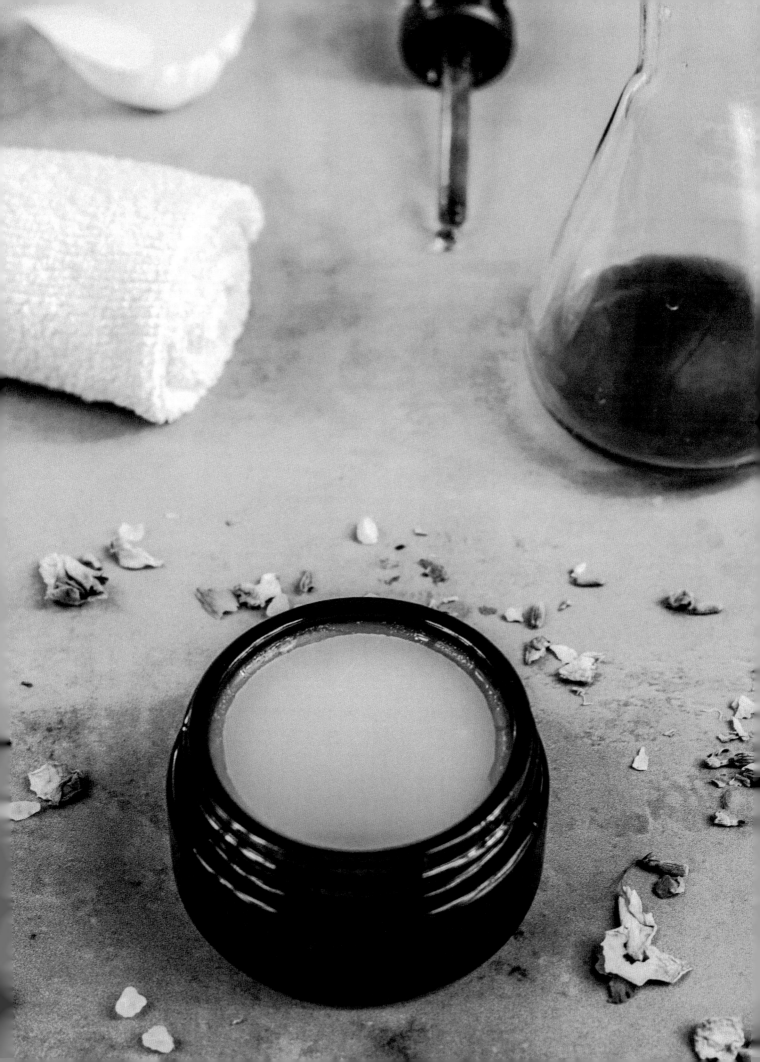

Trust

Trust is especially good for the greasy and greasy/sensitive skin type with a tendency to impurities and clogged pores. It is also good for you who needs to reduce perfectionism and boost your self-esteem. You are doing well enough.

SKIN TYPE

Our Trust Balm contains a cleansing, soothing, uplifting, anti-inflammatory and cooling aromatherapeutic blend of blue tansy, yuzu, frankincense, blue cypress and neroli.

INGREDIENTS

15g	kokum butter
15g	sheabutter
15g	squalane
5g	Ricinus oil or castor oil
5	drops of rosemary CO2 extract
5	drops (approx.) alkanet root extract
3	drops neroli
2	drops frankincense
1	drop blue cypress
2	drops blue tansy
6	drops yuzu

SUPPLIES NEEDED

- Digital scale, weighing down to 1 gram

- 2 small glass measuring cups or bowls or stainless-steel bowls (available in our webshop)

- A chocolate melter or just a bowl for a water bath

- 1 mixing utensil or a small whisk

- 1 tea filter

- 1 50ml jar in dark glass

PROCEDURE

Follow the instructions from the "Bestseller Facebalms" section. Page 66.

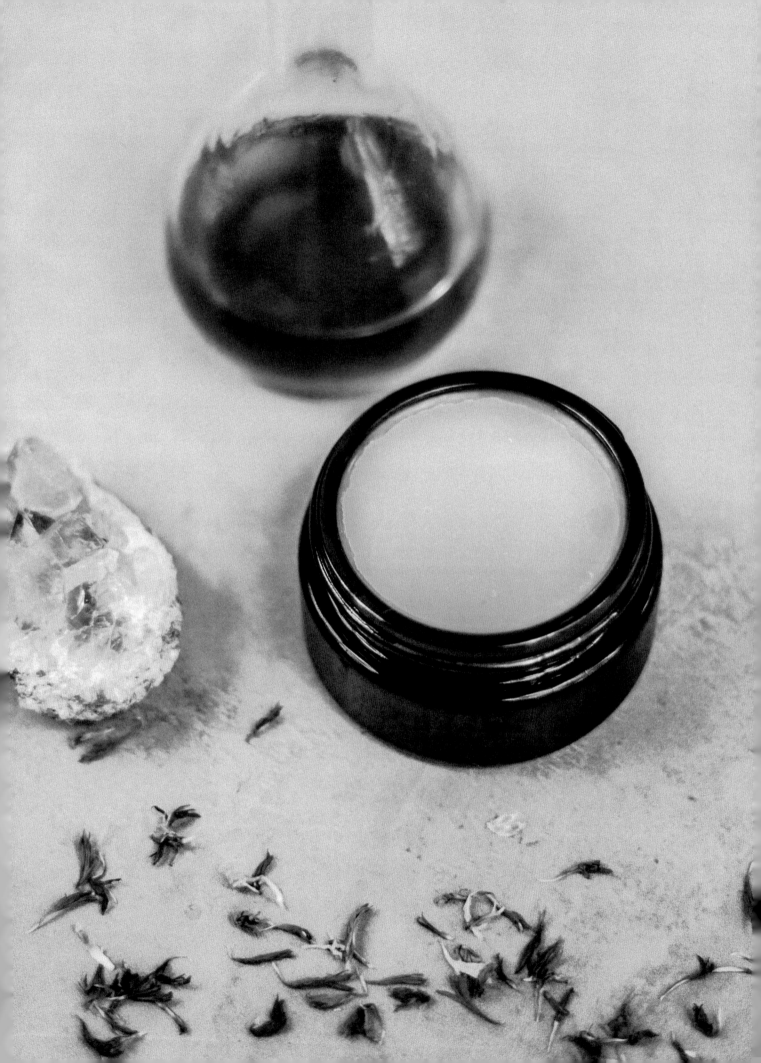

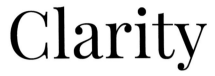

Clarity

Clarity works especially well on the hyperallergic skin or on the skin during pregnancy. It is for you who needs clarity and focus in a world filled with too many choices, opportunities and requirements. It applies to you if you are going through a new life transformation and need to gather yourself, your thoughts and energy somewhere. Peace is a state of mind that you access through breathing.

SKIN TYPE

Our Clarity Balm contains a healing, protective, soothing and mild essential oil-free mixture for those who do not tolerate or want essential oils. Instead, it contains the extract of chamomile and vanilla which mildly calm the skin and mind.

INGREDIENTS

15g   kokum butter

15g   sheabutter

20g   squalane

5g   Ricinus oil or castor oil

5   drops of rosemary CO_2 extract

5   drops vanilla CO_2 extract

3   drops chamomile CO_2 extract

SUPPLIES NEEDED

- Digital scale, weighing down to 1 gram

- 2 small glass measuring cups or bowls or stainless-steel bowls (available in our webshop)

- A chocolate melter or just a bowl for a water bath

- 1 mixing utensil or a small whisk

- 1 tea filter

- 1 50ml jar in dark glass

PROCEDURE

Follow the instructions from the "Bestseller Facebalms" section. Page 66.

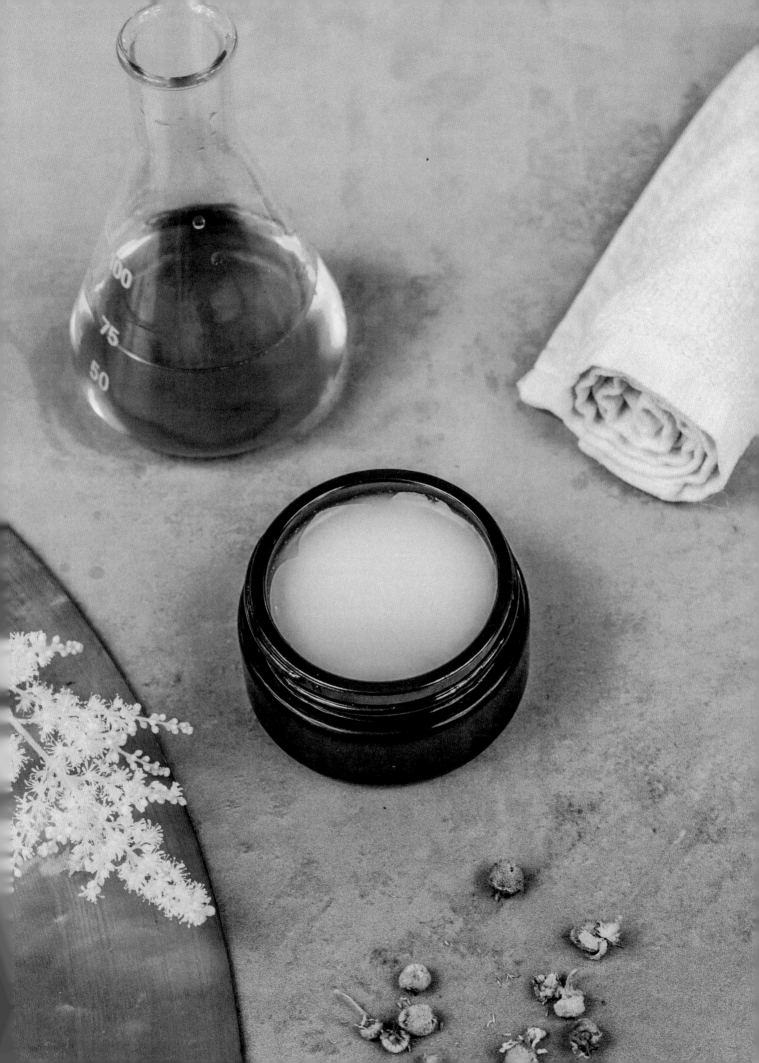

Freedom

Freedom is especially good for combination skin, and for the freedom lovers and pleasure seekers who often get stuck in duties, work overtime and a hyperactive brain. It helps you get out of your head, into the body and home to your heart, so you can breathe easy and embrace life full og adventure, love and freedom. There is only one version of you, so be it 100%.

SKIN TYPE

Our Freedom Balm contains a balanced, renewing and stimulating aromatherapeutic blend of ginger lily, vetiver, viola, green mandarin and jasmine. These ingredients balance skin's sebum production, cleans and stimulates skin regeneration.

INGREDIENTS

15g	kokum butter
15g	sheabutter
10g	squalane
10g	hemp oil
5	drops rosemary CO2 extract
4	drops ginger lily + vetiver
4	drops viola
3	drops jasmine
3	drops clary sage
4	drops green mandarin

SUPPLIES NEEDED

- Digital scale, weighing down to 1 gram
- 2 small glass measuring cups or bowls or stainless-steel bowls (available in our webshop)
- A chocolate melter or just a bowl for a water bath
- 1 mixing utensil or a small whisk
- 1 tea filter
- 1 50ml jar in dark glass
- approx. 2 drops of azulene extract

PROCEDURE

The combination of hemp oil and azulene makes your facebalm green. Pukka's hemp oil is of the best quality and has a deep green color. Use the azulene extract to adjust the color so you get the shade of green that makes you the happiest.Follow the instructions from the "Bestseller Facebalms" section. Page 66.

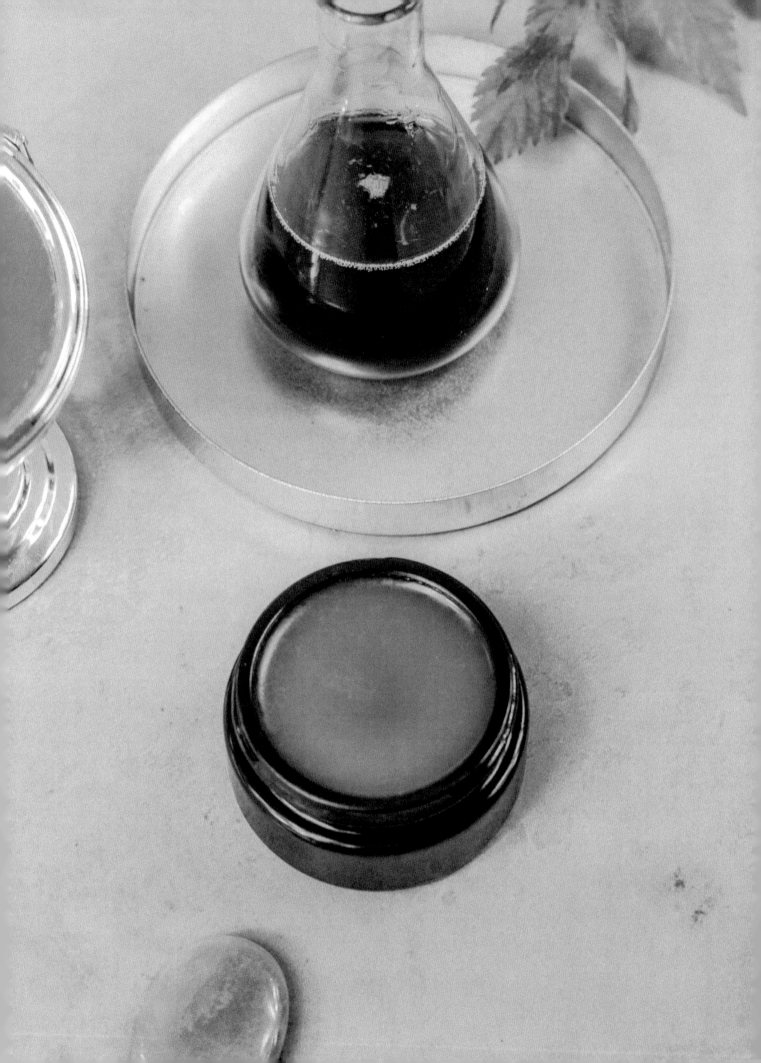

Multi-purpose Facebalm

Your facebalm can be used for much more than just a lubricant for your Gua Sha massage. It is excellent as extra protection under your favorite cream, as a replacement for day and night cream and as a cleansing balm.

GET THE MOST OUT OF YOUR FACEBALM

How to use your facebalm in the morning

In the mornings, you can splash a little water on your face and use a soft washcloth during your morning shower, followed by a small amount of facebalm on damp skin.

If your skin feels dry after a short period of time, then apply your facebalm two times. Start by massaging a thin layer into the skin, wait for one minute, and apply another thin layer. Always apply your facebalm on damp skin. This makes the balm penetrate deeper and faster into the skin, while capturing the moisture from the skin's surface, so your skin feels "plumper" longer.

The first layer of facebalm penetrates deep into the skin, where the essential oils immediately begin to repair and renew the skin.

The second layer of facebalm seals the skin barrier so it can keep moisture in and irritants, pollution and bacteria out.

TIP: Facebalm can be used under the eyes and on the lips for extra night care.

How to use your face balm in the evening

You probably already clean your skin, so why not make it extra luxurious? Enjoy the two minutes you use to wash the day off. Tanja's Aunt of 70 has always spent 30 minutes on "making herself beautiful for the night", and the result can be seen today. She does not have a wrinkle and her skin is moisturized and well kept.

We´re not saying you need to spend 30 minutes on your skin every night. But we are saying "Make the most of the time you spend on yourself by doing it with a mindset of self-love rather than obligation" Enjoy the fragrance of your facebalm as you massage it into your skin. Feel the temperature of the water, the heat of the steam and the texture of the washcloth while you wash and massage the day away.

Appreciate your skin while cleansing it and thank it for taking care of you. The skin barrier is an active part of your immune system, and helps you stay healthy every day.

HOW TO USE THE FACEBALM

- Start by filling the sink, a quarter full, of hot water, but not so hot that you burn yourself.

- Put your washcloth in the water while you massage your facebalm into the skin.

- Take a small pea-sized amount of facebalm with a spatula or the tip of your Gua Sha. Avoid putting your fingers into the balm because of bacteria.

- Rub your hands together to melt the facebalm and release the fragrance molecules.

- Place your hands in front of your nose and close your eyes. Take 10 deep breaths, so the aromatherapy can start its effect on you.

- Massage the balm well into the skin with circular movements. Spend extra time in areas where the pores tend to clog, such as the nose, chin and forehead.

- When you have massaged the balm well into the skin, remove the washcloth from the water, wring it gently and lay the hot washcloth over your face to steam the skin. Let it sit there while you take some deep breaths. If you have very sensitive skin or rosacea, it may not feel good to steam your skin. Do what feels best for you.

- Massage your skin with the washcloth in circular movements so that you thoroughly remove the facebalm.

Repeat the whole process If you have worn makeup or your skin doesn´t feel completely clean. After cleansing your skin, splash cold water on your face and apply a small amount of facebalm as night cream.

NOW YOU'RE READY TO PERFORM YOUR GUA SHA FACIAL.

"The skin barrier is an active part of your immune system, and helps you stay healthy every day. Symptoms reflect how your body and mind are feeling. So, thank your skin and say you're ready to listen now."

TIP
You will find all the ingredients and packaging for our facebalms in our shop honest-beautytalks.org.

Body Gua Sha

Body Gua Sha massage is traditionally used in Chinese medicine to prevent pain and cellulite deposits. You can easily perform the same techniques at home.

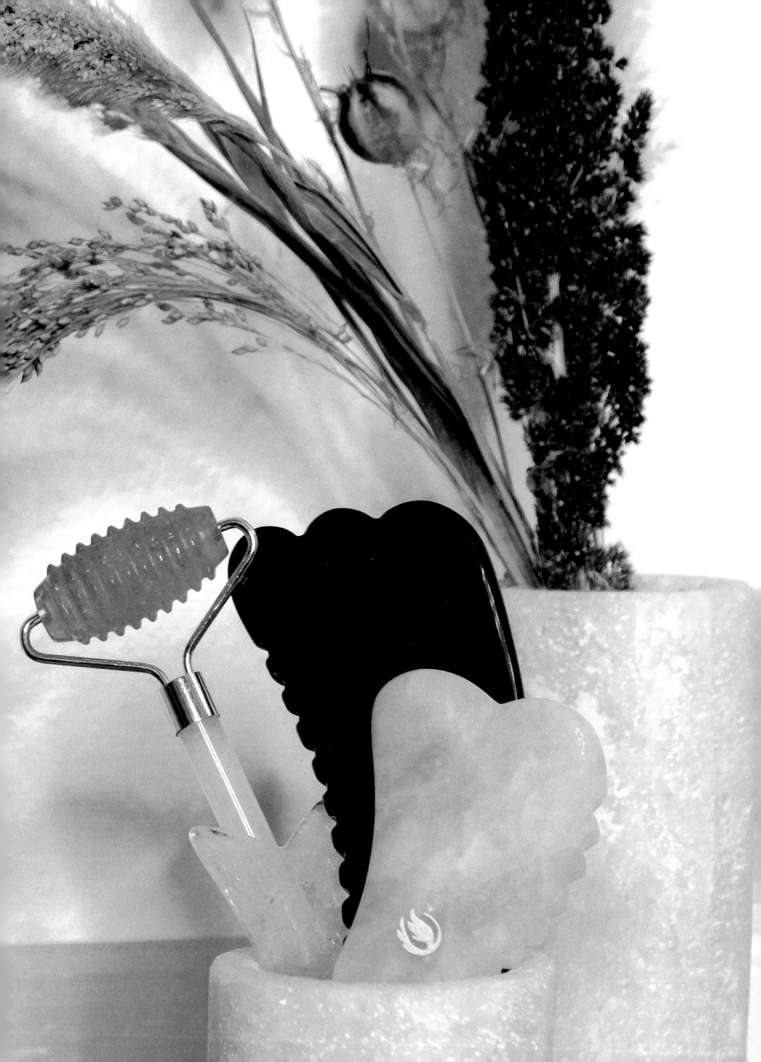

Scrape away your Cellulite

If you are like 90% of us women, then you are familiar with the little bumps, peaks and valleys on your thighs. And you want to smooth them out, right?

We are not saying that we all should be perfectly airbrushed and that cellulite is dangerous, but we would LOVE to shed some light on some of the myths surrounding cellulite. Our intention with this chapter is to focus on how to take loving care of cellulite through gua sha massage and other holistic measures. And kill some stubborn myths by the way we see so many cellulite quick fixes and training programs telling us that we just have to train our way out of cellulite, but honestly has that ever worked for you? We get that you might be frustrated, and the last thing we want is for you to make another failed attempt. That's why we created this body gua sha guide.

In this guide we will share with you, the truth about cellulite and how you can massage, think, breathe and gracefully move past cellulite for good. This is not a quick fix. It will take daily commitment. But we promise it will feel great. You will feel great! And you will look forward to your daily me-time. Here is what you can expect from this program targeting bumps and sagging skin through gua sha massage with our specially designed crystal gua sha tools.

HOW GUA SHA MASSAGE REDUCES CELLULITE

As you begin to release tension and break up facia adhesions with the gua sha tool, you increase blood flow in the skin so that more nutrients enters the skin and waste leaves the skin. It's through blood - as in increased blood flow, that collagen and elastic is delivered to the skin, which firms and tightens skin over time. In addition, you can use the body gua sha massage if you have tense muscles and need extra relaxation.

In this guide, we provide you with a holistic and sustainable treatment of cellulite. The recipes and techniques you find here are proven over the last 3 years, so we know that they work and that you will see results if you put in the effort. Poor diet, poor hydration, lack of movement, weak lymph & blood circulation, suppressed emotions and unresolved anger can all contribute to the accumulation of toxins in the connective tissue and stagnant energy, which causes cellulite and sagging skin. That's why it's so important to take a holistic approach to eliminate the cause of cellulite.

The gua sha techniques alone can definitely reduce cellulite, but if you don't change the circumstances that cause the accumulations, then you need to do the gua sha massage regularly to keep it away. We give you both options in this challenge; The tools to work with the cause as well as gua sha techniques to reduce the symptom. It'is entirely up to you whether you only choose one or decide to go all in.

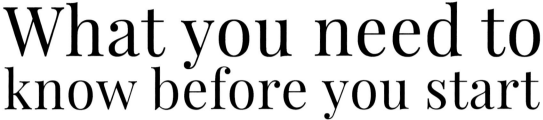

What you need to know before you start

- You may experience some bruising when you start to break up fascia adhesions with the gua sha techniques. Even though it doesn't (and shouldn't!!) hurt to do the gua sha massage. This is quite normal and actually a sign you have worked in the right place! Just don't "chase" bruises, slow and gentle will get you just as far as hard and intensive (which requires much longer rest periods).

- You may feel overwhelmed in the beginning, but remember that 5 min. every other day is better than nothing at all and you will still see results. They just come a little later.

- Results take time! This is not quick fix. It has taken many years to accumulate cellulite and it will also take time to release it. But in a year from now, you wish that you had started today. So just start. Grab your gua sha and start with baby steps today.

- If you tend to get varicose veins and broken blood vessels easily, then move forward slowly and use very light pressure with the gua sha. If you can tolerate body massage without aggravating your symptoms, you can also tolerate gua sha. Gua sha SHOULDN'T HURT. It should feel like apleasant in-depth massage. If it hurts, make it even gentler and slower until the tensions and accumulations dissolve.

Benefits of regular Gua Sha Body Massage

- Reduce cellulite
- Improves blood circulation
- Improves lymphatic drainage
- Promotes a healthy vital glow to the skin
- Promotes skin renewal
- Improves muscle tone by breaking up fascia adhesions causing restricted blood flow to the muscles.

- Gives you softer, smoother and firmer skin.
- Reduces pain, tension and accumulation of cellulite
- More flow and energy in the body
- Less tension and pain
- Relaxed sensation in the body
- Increased body awareness

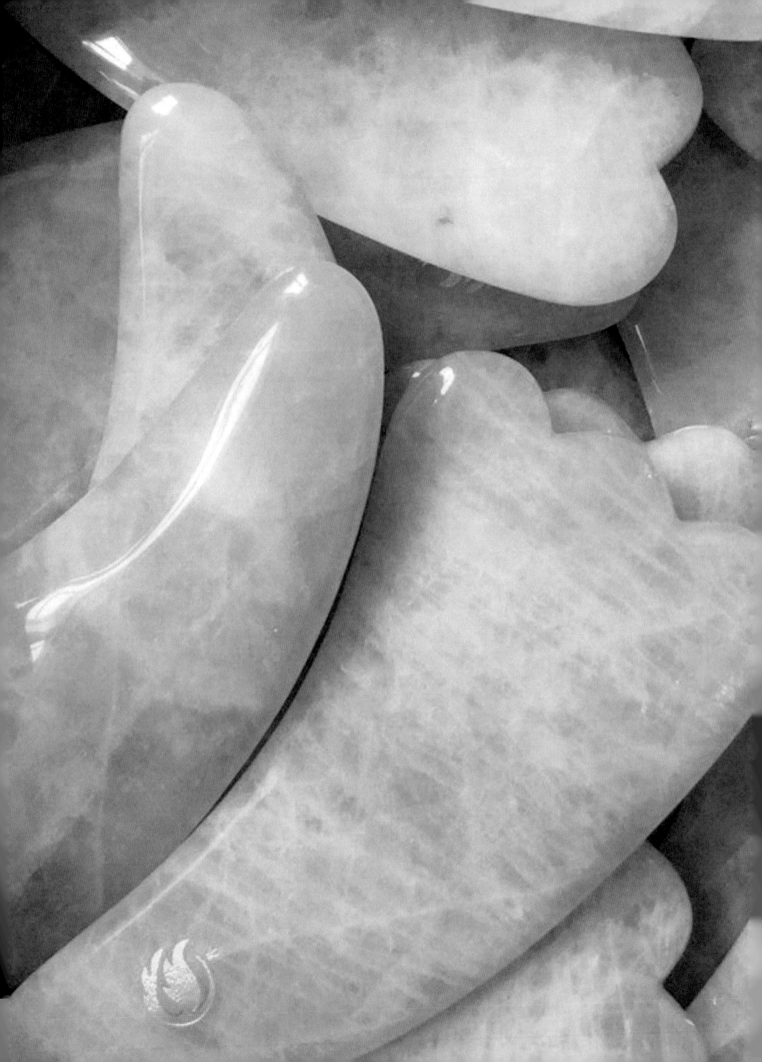

What you need to get started

- A body gua sha with smooth side such
  (as our sodalite, rhodonite or rainbow fluorite xl body gua sha)

- A textured gua sha such
  (as our SHAPE body gua sha in rose quartz or obsidian)

- Your favorite body oil

- 10 mins a day for gua sha massage

The cellulite program is not for you, if you:

- *Are pregnant*
- *Are sick*
- *Are sunburned*
- *Have fever*
- *Have swollen lymph nodes*
- *Have damaged skin*

- *Have fungus or wounds*
- *Got skin cancer*
- *Got inflammation*
- *Easily bruise and leaves permanent damage to blood vessels.*

How fit is your fascia?

Before you start our cellulite programme, you need to identify your cellulite type(s). You do this by taking the "pinch" test developed by Ashley Black Guru. It's normal to have a mix of types in different areas of the body. Use this test to identify your type in you chosen areas and do the test every month to check your progress. Remember to write it down so you can track your results. You can either use the chart to the right and/or the drawing on the next side. Keep in mind that the results in the first few months are most likely subtle and not visible to the eye. But you will feel the difference in your tissues when you repeat the pinch test. This exercise will help you see the results before you can see them on before / after pictures.

If you can lift up the skin and grab 0.5 cm of skin without feeling any pain you have healthy fascia tissue in that area.

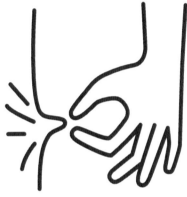

TYPE 1

If you can lift up the skin and grab 1-2 cm and it feels like there are small grains under the skin, you have cellulite type 1.

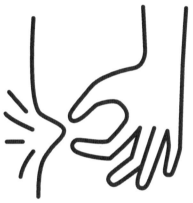

TYPE 2

If you can lift up the skin and grab 1-2 cm and it feels like a burning sensation, then you have cellulite type 2.

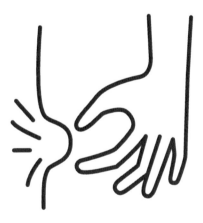

TYPE 3

f you can lift up the skin and get hold of 2+ cm and it feels like gelly / soft you have cellulite type 3.

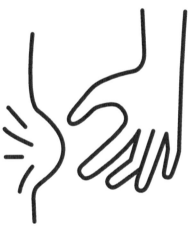

TYPE 4

If you can hardly lift your skin or if you only get large hard lumps, you have cellulite type 4.

Perform the "pinch" test on the areas you wish to keep track of. Insert the result in centimeters in chart below.

RIGHT ANKLE	CM before start	CM 1. måned	CM 2. måned	CM 3. måned
Inside				
Outside				
LEFT ANKLE				
Inside				
Outside				
LEFT CALF				
Outside				
Inside				
RIGHT CALF				
Outside				
Inside				
LEFT THIGH				
Upper part, outside				
Upper part, inside				
Lower part, outside				
Lower part, inside				
RIGHT THIGH				
Upper part, outside				
Upper part, inside				
Lower part, outside				
Lower part, inside				
HIP				
On the side				
WAIST				
Around the belly button				
LEFT ARM				
Forearm, front				
Forearm, back				
Upperarm, front				
Upperarm, back				
RIGHT ARM				
Forearm, front				
Forearm, back				
Upperarm, front				
Upperarm, back				

The Cellulite test

Before you start our cellulite programme, you need to identify your cellulite type(s).
You do this by taking the "pinch" test developed by Ashley Black Guru.

TYPE	PINCH RESULT	HOW IT LOOKS LIKE		CAUSE	FASCIA DEBTH	GUA SHA TREATMENT	TIMELINE RESULTS
1 COTTAGE CHEESE	If you can lift up the skin and grab 1-2 cm and it feels like there are small grains under the skin.	Tiny dimples looking like cottage cheese. Type 1 is the lightest degree of cellulite and the easiest to smooth out.		Restrictions in the outer fascia layers of the connective tissue.	Outermost layer of fascia.	Classic gua sha scraping technique with our Sodalite body gua sha, or the smooth side of our SHAPE body gua sha.	Typically after 1 month when doing gua sha 5-6 times weekly.
2 BUMPS & LINES	If you can lift up the skin and grab 1-2 cm and it feels like a burning sensation,	Larger bumps and lines in the skin.		Restrictions and distortions in the deeper fascia layer of the connective tissue, which cannot be trained or eaten away. But proper hydration helps!	Deeper layers of fascia.	Requires in-depth gua sha massage with side 2 of our SHAPE body gua sha, followed by lymphatic drainage with the sodalite body gua sha or the white jade body gua sha.	Typically after 1-4 months of use 4-5 times weekly.
3 GELLY	If you can lift up the skin and get hold of 2+ cm and it feels like gelly.	The tissue looks bumpy and feels like gelly. There is a lack of muscle tone.		The facia tissue is tangled too tightly around the muscles due to adhesions, making it difficult to build muscle mass.	Deeper layers of fascia.	Requires in-depth gua sha massage with SHAPE's side 2 and side 1 followed by lymphatic drainage with the sodalite body gua sha. Also requires good and proper hydration, diet, yin stretching and strength training.	Typically 6-24 months when used 4-5 times weekly.
4 LARGE LUMPS	If you can hardly lift your skin or if you only get large hard lumps	The skin may look quite smooth, but you can feel large lumps when you squeeze the skin. It can also be seen as "hard" deposits such as "saddle bags"		The facia tissue is completely bond and restricted in all connective tissue layers. Fat, muscle, fluid and accumulations are completely locked.	Deeper layers of fascia.	Requires in-depth gua sha massage with SHAPE's side 4 and 2 followed by lymphatic drainage with sodalite or white jade body gua sha. You may need the "digging technique" with the tip of one of the body gua sha.	Typically 1-2 years when used 4-5 times weekly.

DRAW YOUR CELLULITE TYPES INTO THE FIGURE

We have very visual minds, and we have found that this method really helps increasing body awareness, and of course also helps to see improvements month after month. We think this is a wonderful exercise to check in with the body. Try it out if you want to take this challenge seriously.

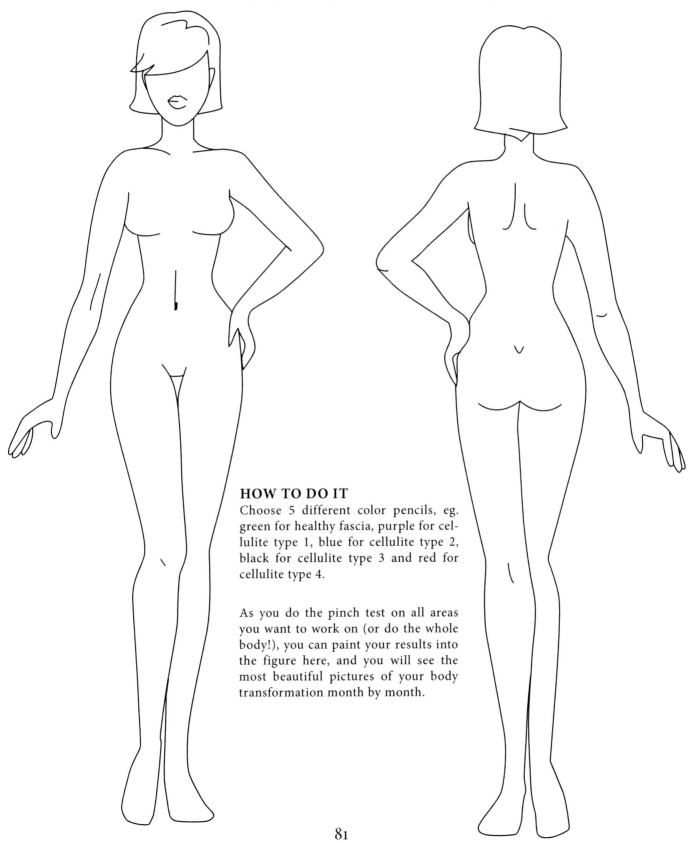

HOW TO DO IT

Choose 5 different color pencils, eg. green for healthy fascia, purple for cellulite type 1, blue for cellulite type 2, black for cellulite type 3 and red for cellulite type 4.

As you do the pinch test on all areas you want to work on (or do the whole body!), you can paint your results into the figure here, and you will see the most beautiful pictures of your body transformation month by month.

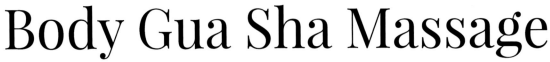

Body Gua Sha Massage

How to perform Gua Sha massage therapy for cellulite.

1. Apply oil to the area you want to work on. Preferably from a spray bottle, as oily fingers are the no. 1 reason why gua sha's break.

2. Using side 1 of your SHAPE Gua Sha tool, scrape light and briskly, but with comfortable firm pressure up and down the area. You can also scrape from side to side but never in circles. From a pain scale from 1-10, where 10 is very painful, you should never exceed a pain level of 3-4. Continue the scraping with side 1 for a few minutes until the surface of the skin is warmed up and has turned slightly pink.

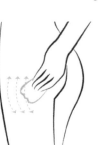

3. Using side 3 of your SHAPE Gua Sha tool or side 1 of any of the XL Body Gua Sha tools, scrape with firm pressure up along the lines of the lymphatic system. So always a long scrape up towards the heart and not up and down as before. Do 10-60 scrapes on the same area before you move on to the next area.

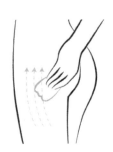

On a scale from 1-10, where 10 really hurts, your level should be around 3-4. I.e. you are working in the connective tissue just below the skin surface. From a scale of 1-10, where 10 really hurts, you should be around a 3-4.

Body Gua Sha Techniques

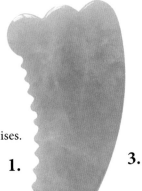

1. Curved pointy side = Smoothes out fascia adhesions, increase blood flow, tightens loose skin. Used for cellulite type 1-3 and warm up for type

2. Waves = Smoothes adhesions in the deeper layers of fascia. Used for cellulite type 4. We recommend you wait 4 weeks before using this technique to avoid too many bruises.

3. The smooth side = Used for classic gua sha scraping technique and final lymphatic drainage. Used for all cellulite types.

4. End = Used for digging into bound up areas of fascia (type 4). Dig into the tissue with small movements and firm pressure to release adhesions and restricted fascia.

Body Gua Sha time overview

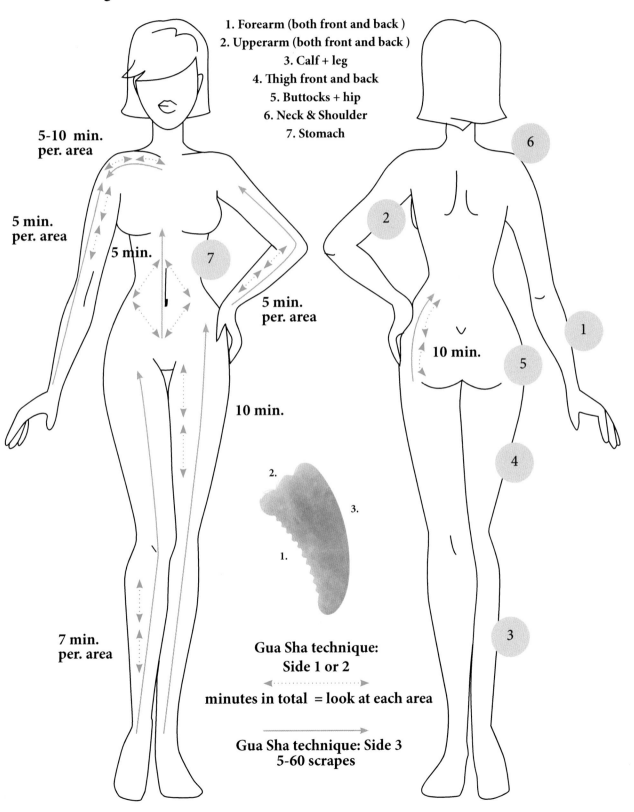

1. Forearm (both front and back)
2. Upperarm (both front and back)
3. Calf + leg
4. Thigh front and back
5. Buttocks + hip
6. Neck & Shoulder
7. Stomach

5-10 min.
per. area

5 min.
per. area

5 min.

5 min.
per. area

10 min.

7 min.
per. area

10 min.

Gua Sha technique:
Side 1 or 2

minutes in total = look at each area

Gua Sha technique: Side 3
5-60 scrapes

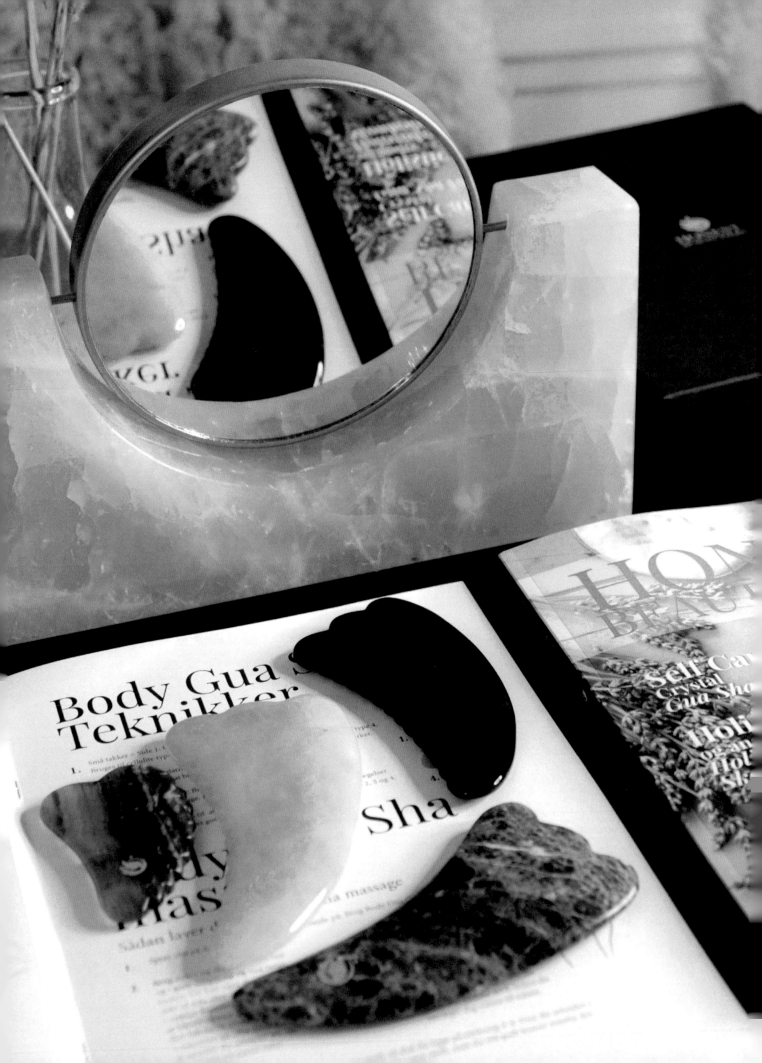

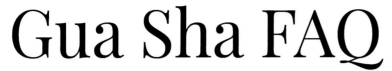

Gua Sha FAQ

AMOUNT OF SCRAPES?

It is important that you continue to scrape the same place at least 5 times and preferably up to 60 (for faster results). It is through repreated scraping that create a vacuum under the skin that draws waste materials up to the surface of the connective tissue, so that it can be removed by the lymphatic system. It must be a firm pressure, but not necessarily hurt. However the tense and stagnant areas will typically a bit. These areas will tend to bruise easily.

LYMPHATIC DRAINAGE?

To avoid or reduce bruising, you can lubricate the area in oil or cream based on arnica. You can get it in most health food stores or in our webshop honestbeautytalks.org. Arnika causes the bruises to disappear significantly faster.

DURATION?

You can do body gua sha daily until you are satisfied with the result. If you get bruises, and the area is too sore, wait a few days until the bruises are gone before you do it again. We recommend you use 5-10 minutes on one body part a day, so that you get the whole body done in one week. It gives the areas plenty of time to recover and you make sure you get to work with your entire fascia system. The fascis system is a holistic system that communicates, which

means that your cellulite on your thighs may well come from tension in the hips, and then you can scrape all you want on your thighs without seeing proper results, before you work on your hips too.

DOES IT HAVE TO HURT TO WORK?

No! From a scale of 1-10, where 10 really hurts, you should be around a 3-4. If you work with the end (side 4) in bound areas, it will be around 4-6 on the scale. Never more!

BRUISES?

The places where there are tension, fascia adhesions and stagnation will typically be more tender and this is also where you can experience bruises when you "break through" the fascia adhesions. So the bruises are really a sign you have worked the right place. It does not mean that you should chase the bruises! Rather make the massage a little lighther, more gentle and take your time. This is a self care practise and something to look forward to. 5-10 mins a day is better than one hour once a week. Do your gua sha while Netflixing or watching @gurujagat lectures. We do!

STANDING UP OR LYING DOWN?

There are no rules, choose what feels most delicious and easy for you. You can do the gua sha in the bed where you can lie down. Then it is easier to work on legs and buttocks and stomach.

WARM OR COLD?

We recommend doing gua sha massage on warm skin. For example, in the sauna or after a bath or exercise. The warmer the skin, the more in depth you can work the connective tissue layers. Another option may be to do it after the tub or in the shower while the skin is still warm and moist. We like to heat up an area with @ leannevenier's Redjuvenator #3 panel, which helps melt away tension and boosts collagen production.

Tip: Be careful not to drop the gua sha in the bathroom and use conditioner instead of oil if you choose to do gua sha in the shower. Then you avoid slippery tiles and clogged drains.

Detoxbalm

The detox balm is the perfect accompaniment to a body Gua Sha massage to combat cellulite. It contains essential oils that improve blood circulation and stimulate lymphatic drainage, thus supporting the detoxifying effect of the Gua Sha massage.

INGREDIENTS

75g shea butter

75g squalene

45g cocoa butter

5 drops of blue cypress

5 drops of helichrysum

5 drops of blue tansy

25 drops of grapefruit

5 drops of linden flower

10 drops of rosemary CO2 extract

SUPPLIES NEEDED

- 200ml jar in dark glass
- 1 small whisk or spoon
- 300ml measuring cup or bowl
- Digital scale, weighing down to 1 gram
- Approx. 10-15 drops of azulenet

PROCEDURE

Start by decontaminating your jar and utensils with rubbing alcohol to remove bacteria.

Weigh the coconut butter and sheabutter in a glass measuring cup and melt over a water bath or in a chocolate melter, until completely melted. Be careful not to overheat the mixture as this will damage the fatty acids. Add squalane, rosemary CO2 extract and azulene. Add as much azulene until you are satisfied with the color.

Make a water bath in a small bowl with ice cubes. Place the cup with the balm mixture in, and hold it firmly, so it doesn´t tip. Stir until the mixture becomes thick and you can draw visible lines in it with a whisk. The color will go from transparent to milky and the texture will get thicker. Pour it onto your 200 ml glass jar before it gets too thick to pour. Screw the lid on tight and place it in the refrigerator for 30 minutes until your balm is completely solid. Your Detox Balm is now ready for use and can last for approx. 9 months with regular storage.

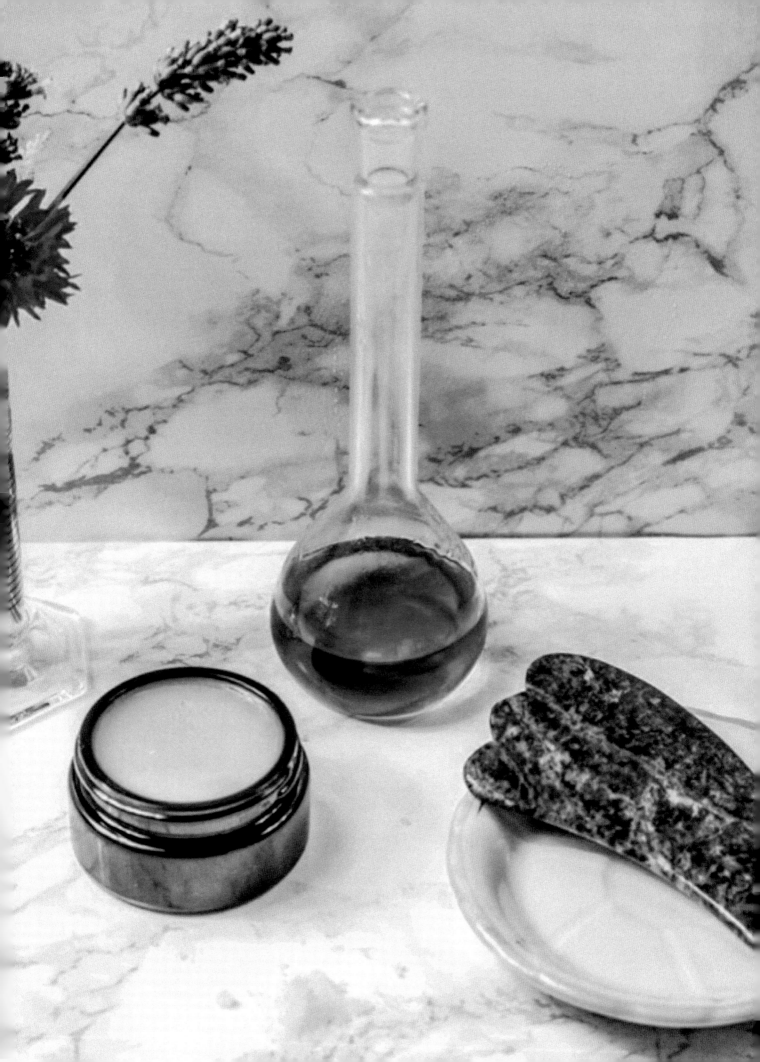

Gua Sha Facials

Our DIY crystal Gua Sha facials are designed to work on your outer beauty and inner health while giving you a "breather" from your everyday life.

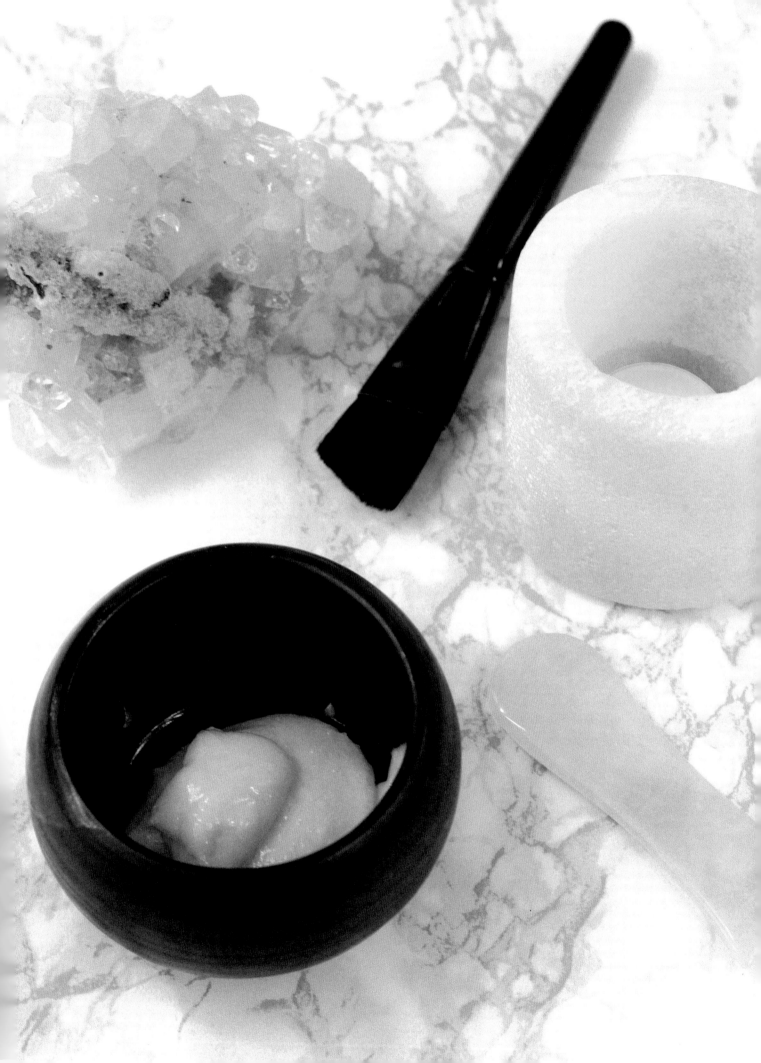

A Good Start

We recommend warming up before your facials, as it makes you more relaxed and enhances the blood flow to your skin.

Our warm-up exercises are excellent if you suffer from tension in your neck.

1. NECK ROLL

Drop your chin toward your chest and slowly roll your head toward one shoulder as you inhale. Roll your head back down toward your chest while you exhale. Proceed to the other side. Repeat the full neck roll 6 times, or as many as you need.

In continuation of the first exercise, gently roll your head all the way around 3 times in each direction. If it feels uncomfortable or you have neck pain, then proceed with the exercise in slow

2. SHOULDER ROLLS

Slowly rotate your shoulders forward, in circles. Repeat the movement backward until the set is complete. Repeat 6 times.

3. SHOULDER RAISES

Lift your shoulders up as you inhale. Hold for a few seconds, then release as you exhale. Repeat 8 times, or as much as you need.

4. SPINE TWISTS

Place your right hand on your left thigh and look over your left shoulder so you feel a stretch in the spine. Repeat in the opposite side.

5. BREATHING

Remember to breathe deeply throughout the entire warm-up. Preferably through the nose.

6. UNDER TIME PRESSURE?

Don´t miss out on your Gua Sha massage just because you don´t have time to do the warm-up. Include the exercises, on the days where you have more time for yourself, as an extra treat.

"Breathing gives you a sense of presence and a peaceful moment to feel and understand your body, so you can achieve greater satisfaction and well-being in your life."

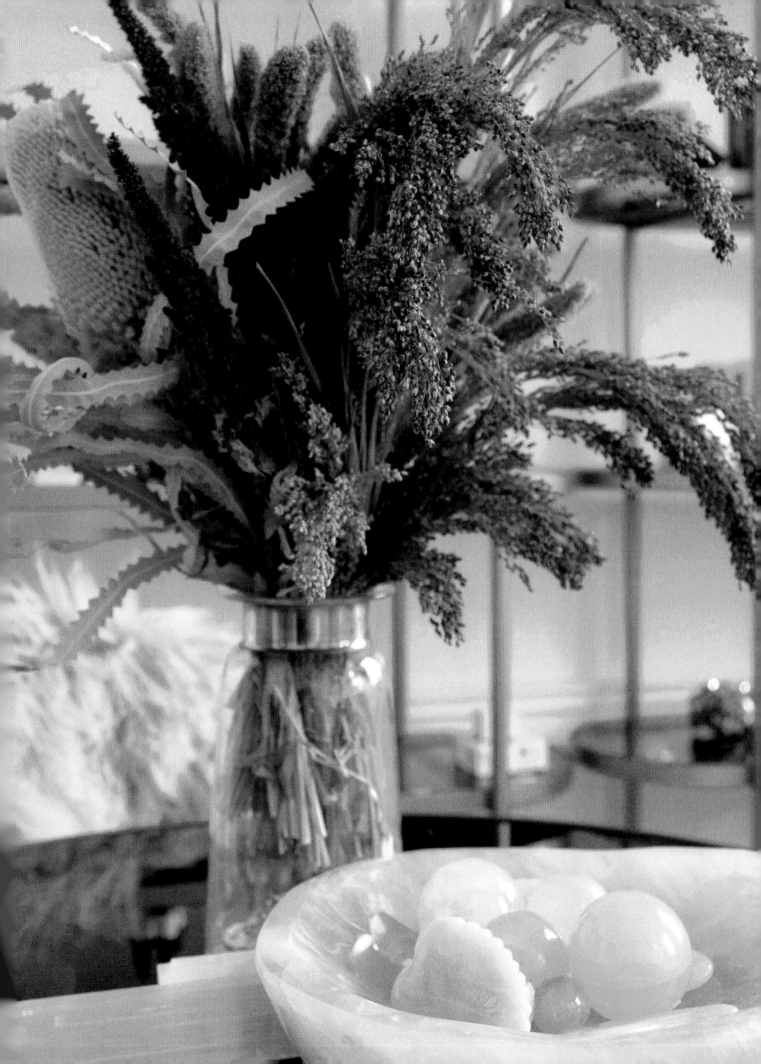

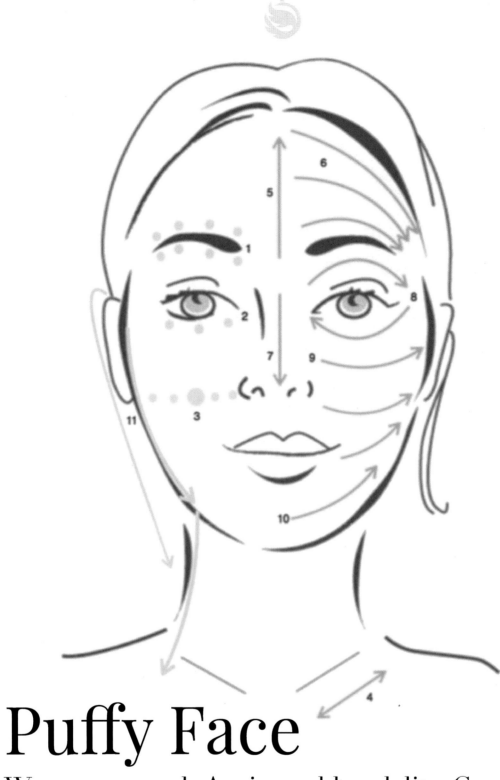

Puffy Face

We recommend: An ice-cold sodalite Gua Sha for the face. This facial should be performed with light pressure and is especially beneficial in the morning when you wake up with a "puffy" face.

STEP 1
Using both hands, pinch your eyebrows with your thumbs and index fingers, drawing them outwards toward the temples. Apply firm pressure along the edge of the eyebrows. Remember to lift your fingers from the skin between compression to protect the fragile skin around the eyes.

STEP 2
Using your fingertips, press the edge of the lower eyelid. (use your index, middle or ring finger). Hold the pressure point while taking a minimum of 2 deep breaths.

STEP 3
Using your thumbs, apply pressure under both cheekbones where they meet your nose. Move firmly under the cheekbone and stop when you reach the tip of the cheekbone (just below the pupil when you look straight out). Hold the pressure point while taking a minimum of 2 deep breaths. This point will typically be sore. Continue out toward the ear.

STEP 4
Open the lymphatic points, by placing your ice-cold Gua Sha, just below the collar bone in each side.

STEP 5
Place the head of the Gua Sha between the eyebrows and scrape up to your hairline. Repeat 10 times with light pressure.

STEP 6
Select one side of the face. Sweep from the top of the center of your forehead (by the hairline) and scrape the Gua Sha head down the hairline to the ear. Repeat 10 times with light pressure. Continue under the previous path with 10 strokes in the same direction. Continue until you have worked through the entire forehead. 3-4 sections should be enough. The final section should be your eyebrows.

STEP 7
Place the tail of the Gua Sha at the top of your nose and scrape down to the tip of your nose. Repeat 10 times with light pressure.

STEP 8
Place the head of the Gua Sha in the temple area. Lightly stroke the area from the temple (outermost part of the eye) and move slowly under the eye toward the nose. Proceed from the inner eye area, up toward the upper part of the eye, and out toward the temple again. Repeat in circles 10 times with very light pressure.

STEP 9
Continue with the Gua Sha head and press lightly from the side of the nose out to the ear. Follow the path just above the cheekbone. Repeat 10 times with light pressure. Continue sweeping, under the previous path, from the side of the nose out to the middle of the ear. Follow the path in the middle of the cheekbone. Repeat 10 times with light pressure. Continue sweeping from the side of the nose, all the way under the cheekbone, until you reach the earlobe. Repeat preferably 10 - 20 times with light pressure. Continue scraping from the corner of your mouth up to the lower part of the ear. Repeat 10 times with light pressure.

STEP 10
Use the wide part of the Gua Sha and sweep from the middle of the chin, along the jawline, and out to the earlobe. Repeat 10 times with light pressure. It can also be beneficial to scrape a few times along the jawline with the tip of the Gua Sha tail.

STEP 11
Stimulate lymphatic drainage by scraping the Gua Sha head from the lower front part of the ear, down the neck, to the collar bone. Repeat 3-5 times, to drain lymphatic fluid, using mild pressure. End the massage, on this side of the face, by stroking the Gua Sha head from behind the upper ear and down the neck with very light pressure, 3-5 times, to drain to the lymph one more time. Lymphatic points are found both in front and behind the ear.

STEP 12
Repeat all steps on the opposite side of the face

EXTRA TIPS

- Treat your skin to an ice-cold water bath. Fill the sink with ice cold water and put your face in it 3-5 times. Or, rub ice cubes on your face.

- Place your Gua Sha in the fridge so it's nice and cold when you're doing your Gua Sha massage.

- You can also cool your face down afterwards with ice-cold crystals.

- Drink fresh celery juice and cucumber as it works as a diuretic.

- Hold back on alcohol and gluten as it increases fluid retention, visible on the skin.

- Remember your two liters of water a day.

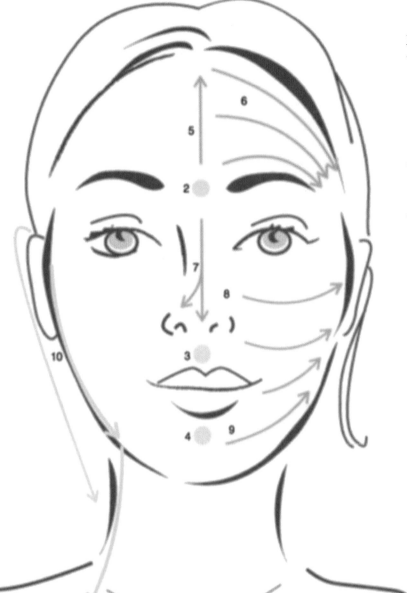

EXTRA TIPS

- Sitali breath - Breathe through a rolled tongue and out through the nose. Do this 26 times each morning and evening. It is a pranayama technique that is known to be anti-inflammatory and cooling.

- Articulate your boundaries to the outside world and stop being a Pleaser.

- Fulfill your basic needs and lower high expectations for yourself. You're doing your best just the way you are.

- Drink strong linden flower tea several times a week

- Strengthen your intestine with fiber and homemade probiotic vegetables.

- Be careful not to over-simulate your skin by using harsh products and avoid soap on your skin. Try cleansing oils instead.

- The pink balm is perfect for your skin type and strengthens the skin barrier. See page 53 under DIY skincare.

Sensitive Skin

We recommend: A rose quartz Gua Sha for the face and the pink Self-Love face balm. This facial should be done with light pressure. Start out slow and gentle if you have very sensitive skin.

STEP 1
Start by opening the "check in" point (under the collar bone). Run your Gua Sha back and forth on the point with medium pressure.

STEP 2
Stimulate the "peace" point between the eyebrows with the tail tip of the Gua Sha by moving it in circular motions. Repeat 5 times to the left and 5 times to the right with medium pressure.

STEP 3
Stimulate the "body / mind" point between the nose and lip with the tail tip of the Gua Sha by moving it in circular motions. Repeat 5 times to the left and 5 times to the right with medium pressure.

STEP 4
Stimulate the "flow" point below the lip with the tail tip of the Gua Sha by moving it in circular motions. Repeat 5 times to the left and 5 times to the right with medium pressure.

STEP 5
Place the head of the Gua Sha on the "peace" point and sweep upward to the hairline. Repeat 5-10 times with light pressure.

STEP 6
Start with one side of the face. Sweep from the top center of your forehead (by the hairline) and scrape the Gua Sha head down the hairline to the upper ear. Repeat 5-10 times with light pressure. If you are very sensitive and turn red easily, then start with 5 times in each area. Continue under the previous path with 5-10 strokes in the same direction. Divide your forehead into 3-4 sections (depending on the size). The final section should be your eyebrows. Next, sweep the Gua Sha from the ear, down the neck, to the "check in" point, just below the collar bone. Remember, very light pressure 3-5 times to drain to the lymph.

STEP 7
Place the center of the tail tip at the top of your nose and scrape down to the tip of your nose. Repeat 5-10 times with light pressure. Use the Gua Sha head and scrape, from the middle of the nose, down the side of the nose. Repeat 5-10 times with light pressure.

STEP 8
Continue to scrape, with the Gua Sha head, from the side of the nose out to the ear. Follow the path just above the cheekbone. Repeat 5-10 times with light pressure. Continue sweeping, under the previous path, from the side of the nose out to the middle of the ear. Follow the path in the middle of the cheekbone. Repeat 5-10 times with light pressure. Continue sweeping from the side of the nose, all the way under the cheekbone, until you reach the earlobe. Repeat preferably 10 - 20 times with light pressure. Continue scraping from the corner of your mouth up to the lower part of the ear. Repeat 5-10 times with light pressure. End this procedure by draining the lymph from the lower ear and down the neck, using with very light pressure 3-5 times.

STEP 9
Place the head of the Gua Sha on the center below the lip and scrape along the jawline. Repeat 5-10 times with light pressure. Use the center of the tail tip, from the middle of the chin, and scrape along the jawline so that you scrape both sides of the jawline at the same time.

STEP 10
Finish this side of the face by scaping the Gua Sha head from the upper part of the ear and down the neck, using very light pressure, 3-5 times. Then sweep behind your ear and down the neck, with very light pressure, 3-5 times to drain to the lymph one more time.

STEP 11
Repeat all steps on the opposite side of the face.

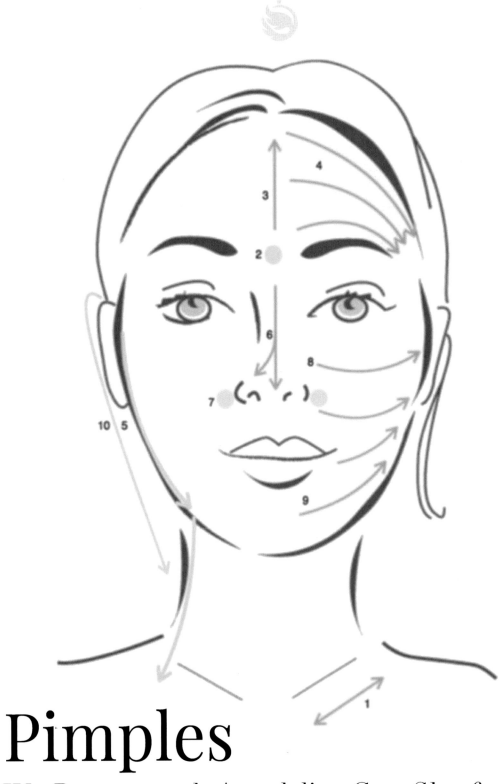

Pimples

We Recommend: A sodalite Gua Sha for the face and the blue Confidence facebalm. This facial should be performed with light pressure. Be sure to clean your Gua Sha with soap after use.

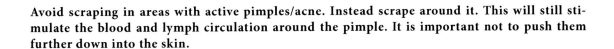

Avoid scraping in areas with active pimples/acne. Instead scrape around it. This will still stimulate the blood and lymph circulation around the pimple. It is important not to push them further down into the skin.

STEP 1
Start by opening the "check in" point (under the collar bone). Run your Gua Sha back and forth on the point with medium pressure.

STEP 2
Stimulate the "peace" point between the eyebrows with the tail tip of the Gua Sha by moving it in circular motions. Repeat 5 times in one direction and 5 times in the other direction with medium pressure.

STEP 3
Sweep the Gua Sha head upwards from the "peace" point to the hairline. Repeat 10-20 times with light pressure.

STEP 4
Start with one side of the face. Sweep from the top center of your forehead (by the hairline) and scrape the Gua Sha head down the hairline to the upper ear. Repeat 10-20 in all. Continue under the previous path with 10-20 strokes in the same direction using light pressure. Work through the entire forehead. Divide your forehead into 3-4 sections (depending on the size). The final section should be your eyebrows.

STEP 5
Scrape from the ear, all the way down the neck to the "check in" point on the collar bone. Remember very light pressure, 3-5 times to drain to the lymph.

STEP 6
Place the center of the tail tip at the top of your nose and scrape down to the tip of your nose. Repeat 10-20 times with light pressure.

STEP 7
Use the Gua Sha tail tip to stimulate the "detox" point on the side of the nose, in circular movements, using light to medium pressure. Repeat 5 times one direction and 5 times in the other direction.

STEP 8
Use the Gua Sha head and scrape, from the middle of the nose, down the side of the nose. Repeat 10-20 times with light pressure. Continue to scrape, with the Gua Sha head, from the side of the nose out to the ear. Follow the path just above the cheekbone, using light pressure. Continue sweeping, under the previous path, from the side of the nose out to the middle of the ear. Follow the path in the middle of the cheekbone. Repeat 10-20 times with light pressure. Continue sweeping from the side of the nose, all the way under the cheekbone, until you reach the earlobe. Repeat preferably 10 - 20 times with light pressure. Continue scraping, with the Gua Sha head, from the corner of your mouth up to the lower part of the ear. Repeat 10-20 times with light pressure. End this procedure by draining the lymph from the lower ear and down the neck, using with very light pressure 3-5 times.

STEP 9
Place the head of the Gua Sha on the center below the lip and scrape along the jawline. Repeat 10-20 times with light pressure. Continue to scrape, with the Gua Sha head, in the same direction, under the previous path on the jawline. Use the center of the tail tip, from the middle of the chin, and scrape along the jawline so that you scrape both sides of the jawline at the same time.

STEP 10
Use the Gua Sha head and scrape down the side of the neck to drain to the lymph. Repeat 3-5 times with very light pressure. Finish this side of the face by scraping the Gua Sha head from behind the ear and down the neck, using very light pressure, 3-5 times to drain to the lymph one more time.

STEP 11
Repeat all steps on the opposite side of the face. Remember to breathe deeply while doing the massage, as to release tension and blockages.

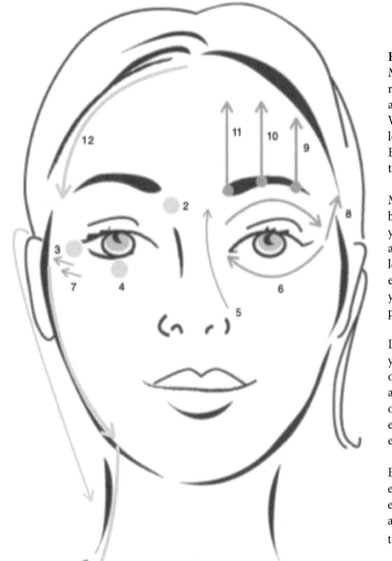

Eye Fitness Exercises

Make sure your head and neck are relaxed and that you are looking at a point straight in front of you. Without moving your head or neck, look to the right as you breathe in. Breathe out as your eyes move back to the center.

Move your eyes to the left as you breathe in and back to the center as you exhale. Inhale and look down and return to center as you exhale. Breathe in and look up and on exhalation, back to center. Close your eyes for 5 seconds and then repeat the exercise 2 times more.

Look straight at a point in front of you. Without moving your head or neck, roll your eyes all the way around. First one way and then the other. Repeat 3 times. Close your eyes for a few seconds between the exercises.

Exercise tones the skin around the eyes, gives life and vitality to the eyes, increases blood circulation and smooths the eyebrows. Helps tired and dry eyes.

Eye Lift

We recommend: An amethyst Gua Sha for the face and your favorite facebalm. Amethyst is often used for eye problems and headaches.

STEP 1

Start by opening the "check in" point just below the collar bone by moving your fingertips in circles on the point. Open both points at the same time.

STEP 2

Press the point, just below where the eyebrows start, near the bridge of the nose. Hold the pressure on both sides of the face at the same time and press firmly for 10-15 seconds. This point is often tender, so you won't be in doubt when you find it.

STEP 3

Press the point on the outer edge of the eye, near the temples, on both sides of the face at the same time, with firm pressure for 10-15 seconds.

STEP 4

Press the point right below the center of the eye, on both sides of the face at the same time, using firm pressure for 10-15 seconds. This point is located on the edge of the lower eyelid, just below the pupil, when looking straight out. (You may notice a small arch where the point is).

STEP 5

Use the edge of the Gua Sha head and scrape from the side of the nose, up the nose, until you reach the eyebrow. Scrape 10 times with medium pressure.

STEP 6

Use the Gua Sha head, to scrape from the outer edge of the eye, located just below the eye, on the soft part. Sweep toward the inner edge of the eye and over the eyelid toward the outer edge of the eye. Continue in circles, 10 times, with very light pressure.

STEP 7

if you have crow's feet: Gently stretch the area with your index finger and long finger. With the other hand, use the Gua Sha head or tail tip and scrape back and forth, or in zigzag motions, over the crow's feet. Repeat 5 times over each line, using light to medium pressure. Skip this step if you don't have crow's feet.

STEP 8

Use the edge of the Gua Sha head and scrape from the edge of the outer eye out to the hairline with medium pressure 10 times.

STEP 9

Use the tip of the Gua Sha tail to stimulate the outer point of the eyebrow (back and forth, up and down and in circles). Now take the edge of the Gua Sha head and scrape from the eyelid / point in a straight line up to the hairline with medium pressure 10 times.

STEP 10

Repeat entire step 9 in the middle of the brow with medium pressure 10 times.

STEP 11

Repeat entire step 10 at the inner point of the eyebrow at the bridge of the nose.

STEP 12

Finish this side of the face by scraping the Gua Sha head from the center of the hairline and down to the temple. Continue down the ear and neck to drain the lymph, 3-5 times with light pressure.

STEP 13

Repeat all steps on the opposite side.

EXTRA TIPS

- End the massage by placing ice-cold crystals (we recommend amethyst) or cucumber slices on your eyes and give yourself a minimum of 5 minutes to lay and relax.

- Get your beauty sleep. Use a sleep mask or sleep in total darkness.

- It can be seen immediately on your eyes if you are dehydrated, so remember at least 2 liters of water every day.

- Face Fitness for the eyes. Remember that you get our online Facegym membership, free of charge, when you buy a Gua Sha crystal at honestbeautytalks.org.

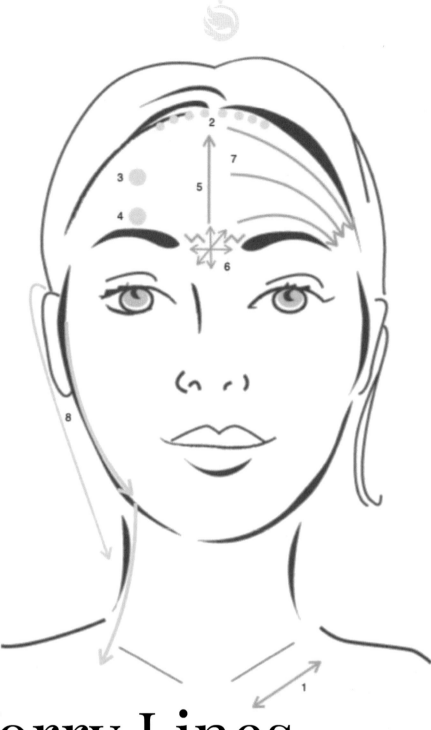

Worry Lines

We recommend: An aventurine Gua Sha for the face and the green Liberty facebalm. Aventurine is for you who needs to let go of your worries and invite adventure into your life instead.

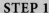

STEP 1
Start by opening the "check in" point just below the collar bone by moving your fingertips in circles on the point. Open both points at the same time.

STEP 2
Use your fingertips from each finger, except your thumb, and place them along the hairline on the forehead. Bend your head forward and hold with medium to firm pressure for at least two deep breaths.

STEP 3
Run your index fingers in circles, toward each other, on the higher points of the forehead, on both sides of the face. Move 10 circles along the hairline, using firm pressure.

STEP 4
Run your index fingers in circles, toward each other, on the lower of the forehead, on both sides of the face. Move 10 circles along the hairline, using firm pressure.

STEP 5
Sweep the Gua Sha head upwards from the "peace" point to the hairline. Repeat 10-20 times with light pressure.

STEP 6
Stimulate the "peace" point, between the eyebrows, with the tip of the Gua Sha tail. Move it in circular motions using light to medium pressure, 5 times in one direction and 5 times in the other direction.
Use the tail tip to make zigzags over the wrinkle(s). Repeat 3-5 times over each line.

If you tend to tense up between the brows, you can use the edge of the Gua Sha head to scrape from the point between the brows and a few centimeters out, in small strokes, using firm pressure 10-20 times. Start with the left brow and scrape up and out 10-20 times. Continue in the middle, up and out, 10-20 times and then toward the right 10-20 times, so that you relax the entire area between the brows. Spend more time on areas where you feel tension.

STEP 7
Start with one side of the face. Use the Gua Sha head and scrape from the eyebrow to the ear, 10-20 times with medium to firm pressure. Then proceed, in the same pattern, on the next line and end on the path at the hairline.

STEP 8
Finally, scrape from your ear and down the neck to the "check in" point below the collar bone. Repeat 3-5 times, using very light pressure to drain to the lymph.

STEP 9
Repeat steps 7 and 8 on the opposite side of the face.

EXTRA TIPS

- Are you in doubt whether you tense the muscle between the brows? A good way to answer that question is to put a piece of tape on your forehead (do this at home or when you sit in front of the computer).

- This can help you become more aware of when you, unnecessarily, tense your forehead. Thus, preventing it next time.

- Always remember to wear sunglasses when the sun is shining.

- The zone between the brows is said to be related to the liver. Therefore, always support your live with a little extra care. We recommend giving your liver extra love and care by drinking dandelion juice 2-3 times a day (before a meal).

- If there is something that worries or frustrates you, then remember that 90% of your worries never turn into anything. If you can´t do anything about it, let it lie.

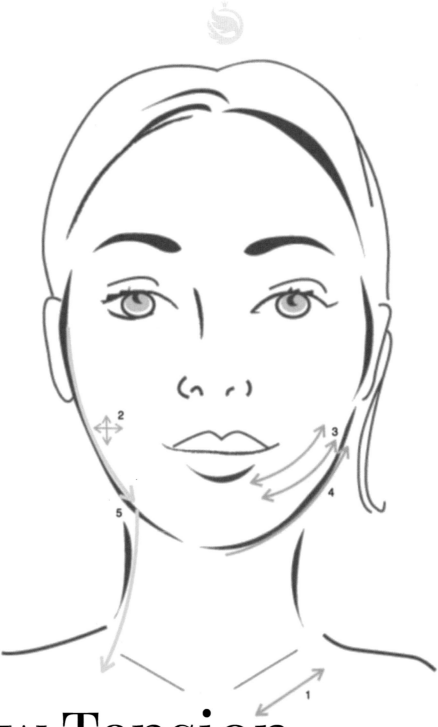

Jaw Tension

We recommend: One of our body Gua Sha'er. You can choose between soda body, rose quartz body or obsidian or rose quartz SHAPE Gua Sha. Also, remember your favorite facebalm.

STEP 1

Start by opening the "check in" point just below the collar bone by moving your fingertips in circles on the point. Open both points at the same time.

STEP 2

Find your chewing muscle by clenching your teeth together and see the muscle contract. Open your mouth slightly so your jaw feels relaxed. Massage the muscle with 2 or 3 fingers in large circular movements, applying medium to firm pressure, for at least 30 seconds.

STEP 3

Use the "scalloped" end of the body Gua Sha to move, back and forth, over the jaw muscle. Hold the Gua Sha in a horizontal position and place it on the muscle. Scrape back and forth over the muscle while relaxing your jaw and keeping your mouth slightly open. You can massage the whole jaw area in this way. Continue until your jaw feels relaxed for a minimum of 30 seconds and up to 2 minutes.

STEP 4

Use the curved end of the Gua Sha and scrape from the mouth to the ear, so you get the whole jaw in one stroke. Scrape 10-20 times, back and forth, with light pressure.

STEP 5

Finish this side of the face by scaping the Gua Sha from the lower ear and down the neck, using very light pressure, 3-5 times to drain to the lymph.

STEP 6

Repeat all steps on the opposite side of the face.

EXTRA TIPS

- Think about what you suppress during the day, which you don´t express. We recommend expressing your opinion out loud.

- Notice how you, unconsciously, clench your teeth throughout the day.

- Refrain from chewing gum

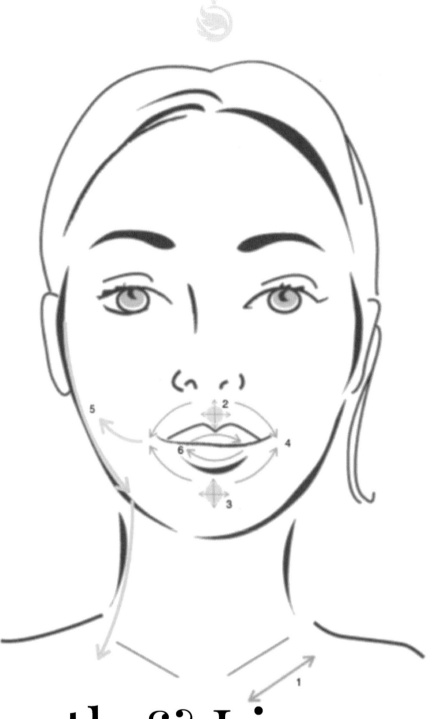

Mouth & Lips

We recommend: Your favorite face Gua Sha and facebalm. Use the Gua Sha made of mountain crystal if you have dry or chapped lips.

STEP 1

Start by scraping back and forth on the "check in" point in both sides.

STEP 2

Stimulate the "body / mind" point over the lip with one of the tail tips on the Gua Sha. Move back and forth, op and down, and in circles on the point.

STEP 3

Stimulate the "flow" point below the lip with one of the tail tips on the Gua Sha Move back and forth, op and down, and in circles on the point.

STEP 4

Start on one side and scrape the Gua Sha head along the upper lip line, using medium pressure, 10-20 times. Emphasize on areas where you feel a tension or where you have lines and continue to scrape back and forth. Repeat on the lower lip line.

STEP 5

Finish this side of the face by scaping the Gua Sha from the lower ear and down the neck, using very light pressure, 3-5 times to drain to the lymph.

STEP 6

You can also scrape directly on your lips to stimulate blood circulation and give a "plump" effect.

STEP 7

Repeat steps 4 and 5 on the opposite side.

EXTRA TIPS

- Treat your lips to a good lip balm but avoid lip balm with mineral oils as they dry your lips and make your them dependent on constant moisturizing.

- Protect your lips from the sun, wind and cold temperatures.

- Avoid smoking and excessive use of straws.

- Use a lip mask made of honey a couple of times a week. Leave the honey on for 10 minutes.

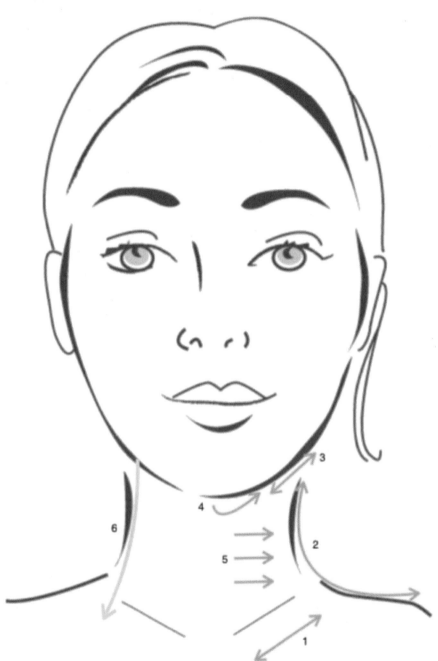

Neck & Jawline

We recommend: Your favorite face Gua Sha and facebalm.

STEP 1
Start by scraping back and forth on the "check in" point in both sides.

STEP 2
Start on one side and scrape up and down with the Body Gua Sha in long strokes on the side of the neck and around the neck.

STEP3
Continue in the same side and scrape back and forth under the jaw.

STEP 4
Scrape under the chin

STEP 5
Start at the base of your neck and work slowly upward, concentrating on the lines along the way. Scrape carefully with an upward sweep or pinch the skin gently. Remember to be extra gentle here as our skin on the neck can be very thin and sensitive.

STEP 6
Finish by scraping down the neck 3-5 times, using light pressure, to drain to the lymph.

STEP 7
Repeat all steps on the opposite side.

EXTRA TIPS

- Avoid turkey neck! Look up instead of looking at your phone all the time! Remember a little screen detox every now and then.

- Make sure your skin care routine doesn´t stop at the jawline. Remember to moisturize the all the way down the neck.

- Face Fitness for the neck. Remember that you get free membership when you purchase a Gua Sha crystal at honestbeautytalks.org.

FACE FITNESS FOR THE NECK

EXERCISE 1
Look straight ahead and place your fingertips on your neck. Let your fingers slide down to the collar bone, while slowly bending your head backwards. Feel a stretch in your neck.

Repeat 2 times more.

While holding the last stretch, with your head tilted back, lift your chin as high as you can and turn the corners of your mouth downward. Keep the stretch for 4 long breaths.

Exercise tones the neck and jaw area and minimizes saggy skin.

EXERCISE 2
Place the palm of your hand under your chin (like a shelf). Place the other hand under your elbow to support the arm holding your chin. Press your hand underneath your chin to provide gentle resistance as you push them toward one another. Hold for 10 seconds.

Repeat 2 times more.

Finish by slapping the skin underneath the chin, alternately with both hands, for 15 seconds. This exercise stimulates collagen and elastin production.

The exercise tightens the skin under the chin, which quickly loses elasticity and becomes saggy.

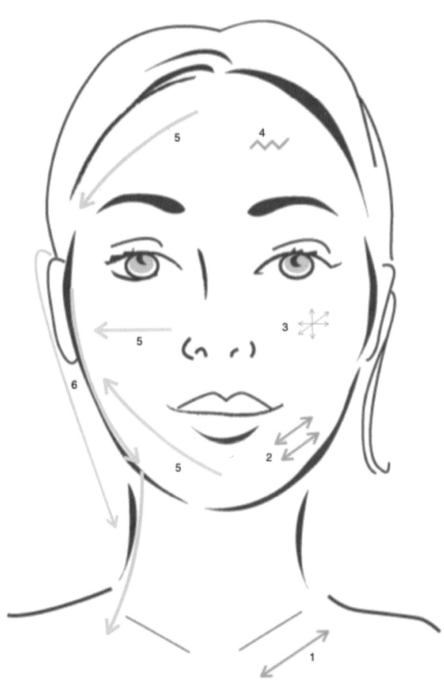

Scar Tissue & Wrinkles

We recommend: Your favorite face Gua Sha and facebalm plus a body Gua Sha or SHAPE Gua Sha.

STEP 1
Start ar the "check in" point, with the Gua Sha head, by scraping back and forth with medium pressure.

STEP 2
Use the "scalloped" end of the body Gua Sha, if you have several acne scars in the jaw area. Start by stretching your skin, gently pulling your skin toward the ear. Scrape the Gua Sha over the scarred area, back and forth, to break down the scar tissue. Use light to medium pressure. Do this for a few minutes, until the area has become slightly red.

STEP3
Select an area with deep scars or wrinkles. Gently stretch the skin with one hand and apply the face Gua Sha with the other hand. Scrape with the head or tail tip up and down, from side to side and diagonally.

STEP 4
Use the tail tip on the face Gua Sha if you have minor or major scarring elsewhere on the face. Scrape in zigzag motions while stretching the skin out with the other hand. It is the same zigzag technique that you use for wrinkles. Continue this for a few minutes, until the area is red. The pressure is medium, but make sure you don´t damage the skin!

STEP 5
Scrape with the back of the body Gua Sha from the middle of the forehead and out to the ear with light pressure in a large stroke, 3-5 times. Then scrape the whole cheek area from the nose to the ear in a large stroke with light pressure, 3-5 times. Finally, scrape the chin and jaw area in one large stroke ,3-5 times, using light pressure.

STEP 6
Finish by draining the lymph, with very light pressure, down the neck 3-5 times. Scrape down, a few times, behind the ear for extra lymphatic drainage.

EXTRA TIPS

- Remember sun protection and wear a sun hat.

- Get lots of antioxidants like green tea and blueberries that help prevent scars and wrinkles.

- Apply good, natural and nutritious oils such as rosehip oil or pure vitamin E oil on new and old scars to help them heal and fade faster.

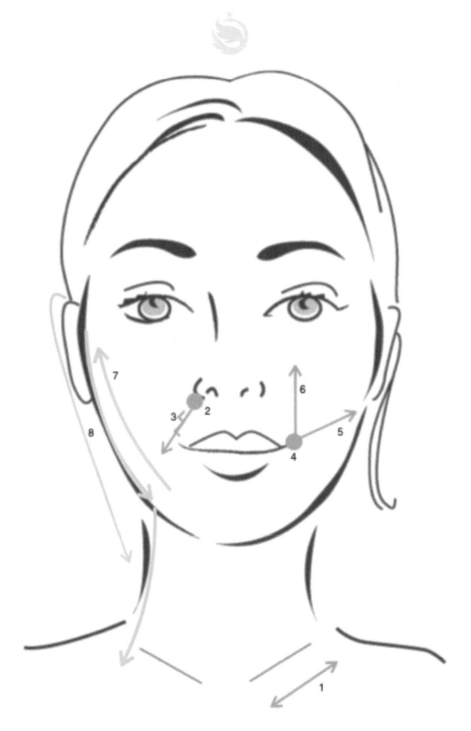

Cheek Lift

We recommend: Your favorite face Gua Sha and facebalm.

STEP 1
Start at the "check in" point, with the Gua Sha head, by scraping back and forth with medium pressure.

STEP 2
Use the Gua Sha tail tip to stimulate the "detox" point on the side of the nose, using light to medium pressure. Scrape up and down, back and forth and in circles clockwise and counterclockwise.

STEP3
Use the Gua Sha head and scrape in a line from the "detox" point and down along the line, starting from the nose. Turn the Gua Sha around and use the tail tip to make zigzags up and down the line. We call this "Zigzag" movement an eraser as it reduces lines and wrinkles.

STEP 4
Use the Gua Sha tail tip to stimulate the point from the corner of the mouth, applying light to medium pressure. Scrape up and down, back and forth and in circles clockwise and counterclockwise.

STEP 5
Scrape in a line with the Gua Sha head from the corner of the mouth and toward the ear (the line is below the cheekbone). Repeat at least 5 times with medium pressure.

STEP 6
Scrape in a line with the Gua Sha head from the corner of the mouth and straight up so you lift the cheek with the Gua Sha. Repeat at least 5 times with medium pressure.

STEP 7
Scrape the whole cheek to the lymph point, using light pressure.

STEP 8
Continue with light pressure to scrape down the front of the ear and down the neck. Finish by scraping from behind the ear and down the neck.

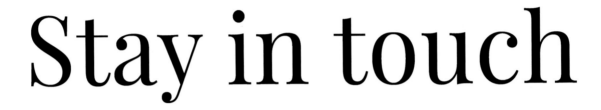

Stay in touch

WE WOULD LOVE TO HEAR FROM YOU!

You can always connect with us on our free Facebook membership group:
http://tinyurl.com/facebookhbt

Or write us an email at care@honestbeautytalks.org

WANT TO LEARN MORE GUA SHA TECHNIQUES?

Remember you get lots of DIY video tutorials when you purchase a beauty tool from our site:
honestbeautytalks.com

We do yearly Gua sha certification courses for professionals. For more info go here:
https://www.honestbeautytalks.com/courses

#CAREFORYOURSELF

Maja & Tanja

Honestbeautytalks.com

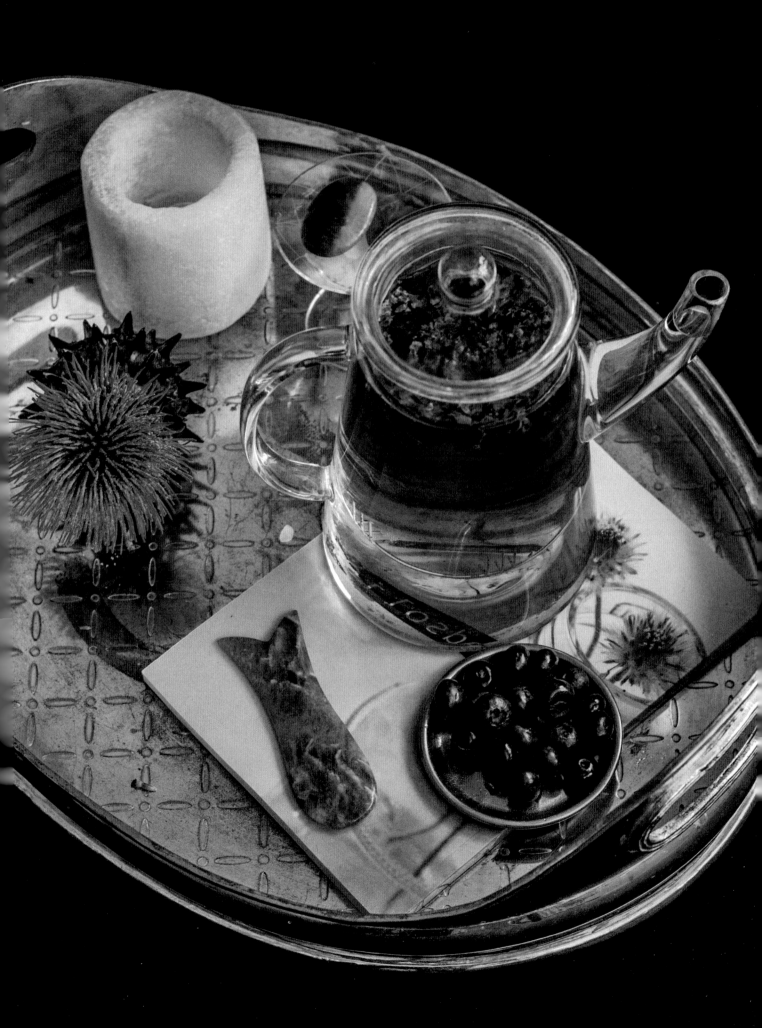

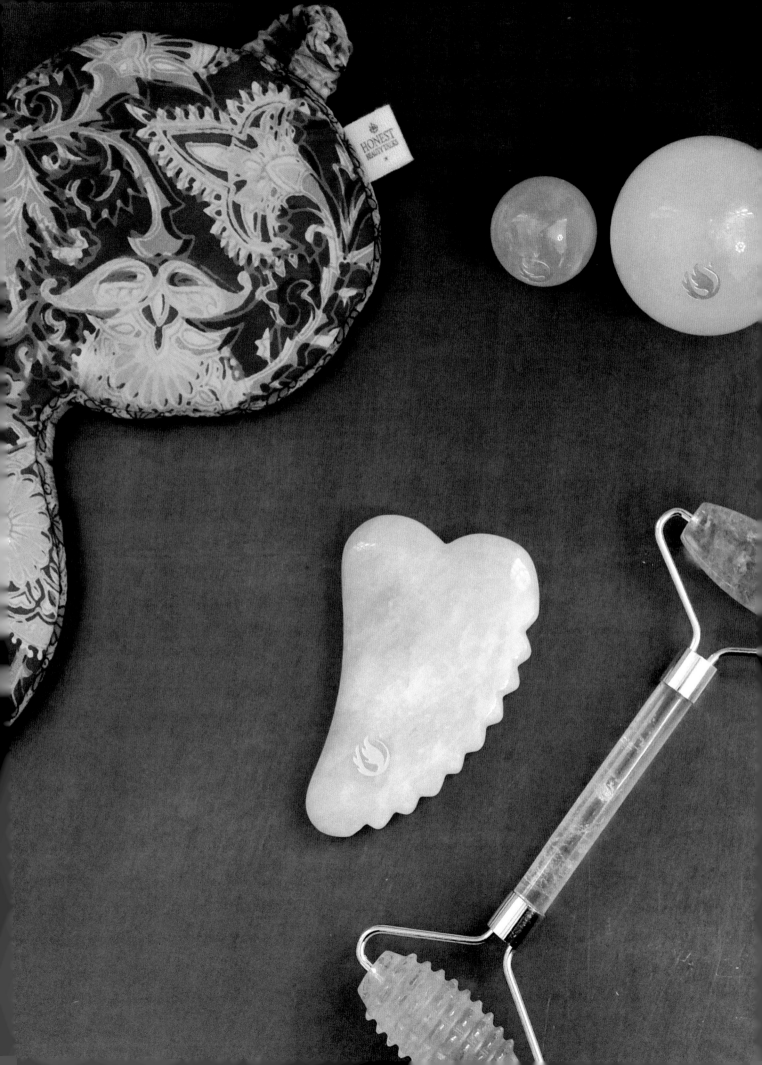

Made in the USA
Las Vegas, NV
27 February 2025

18792912R00071